P9-CQT-076

THE
SWEET
LIFE

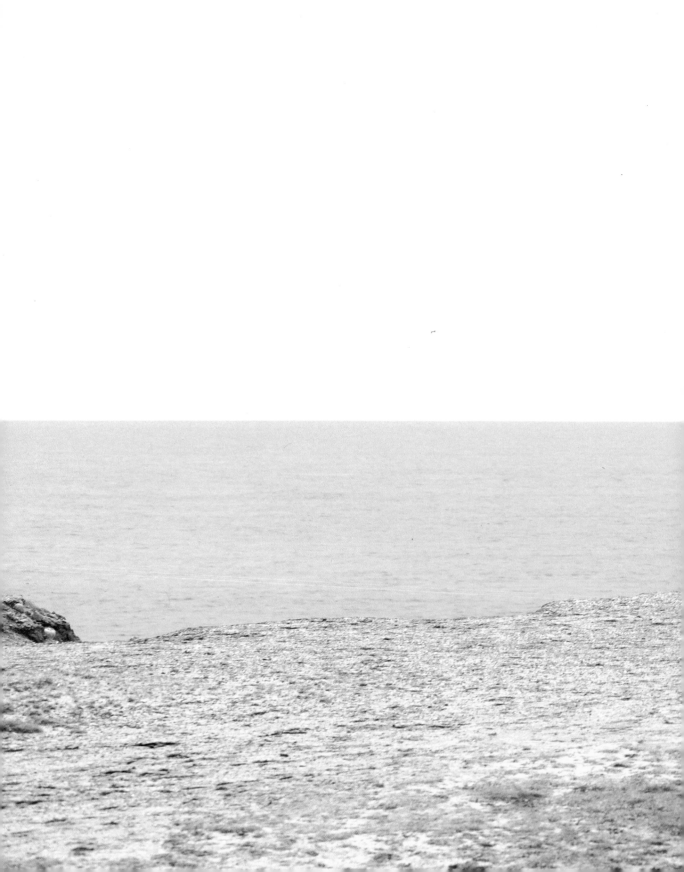

THE SWEET LIFE

Diabetes without Boundaries

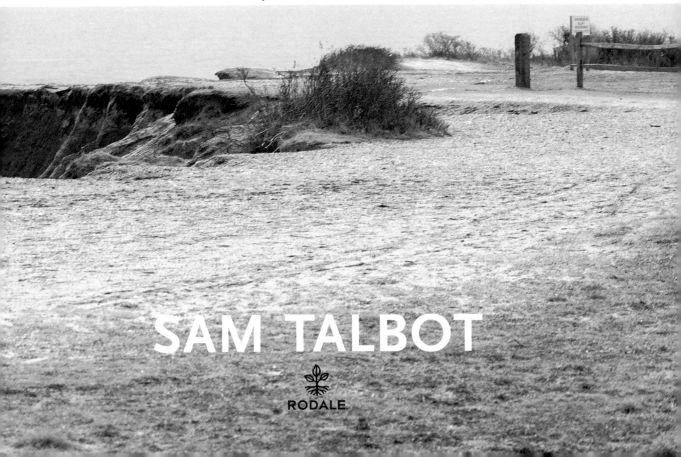

SAM TALBOT

RODALE

© 2011 by Sam Talbot

Principal food photography © 2011 by Tara Donne

All rights reserved. No part of this publication may be reproduced or transmitted in any form
or by any means, electronic or mechanical, including photocopying, recording, or any other information
storage and retrieval system, without the written permission of the publisher.

Rodale books may be purchased for business or promotional use or for special sales.
For information, please write to: Special Markets Department, Rodale Inc., 733 Third Avenue, New York, NY 10017.

Printed in the United States of America
Rodale Inc. makes every effort to use acid-free ∞, recycled paper ♻.

Book design by Emily Anderson and Kara Plikaitis

Lifestyle photography © 2011 by Joe Termini and Sarah Kehoe

Library of Congress Cataloging-in-Publication Data is on file with the publisher.

ISBN-10: 1–60529–095–5 hardcover

ISBN-13: 978–1–60529–095–9 hardcover

ISBN-13: 978–1–60961–459–1 Special Sales Edition

Distributed to the trade by Macmillan

2   4   6   8   10   9   7   5   3   1   hardcover

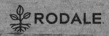

RODALE

We enable and inspire people to improve their life and the world around them.
www.rodalebooks.com

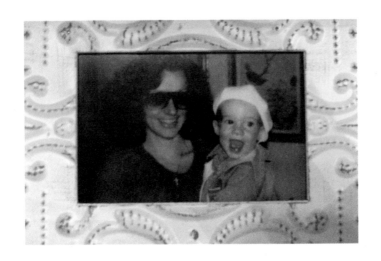

Dear Mama—thanks.

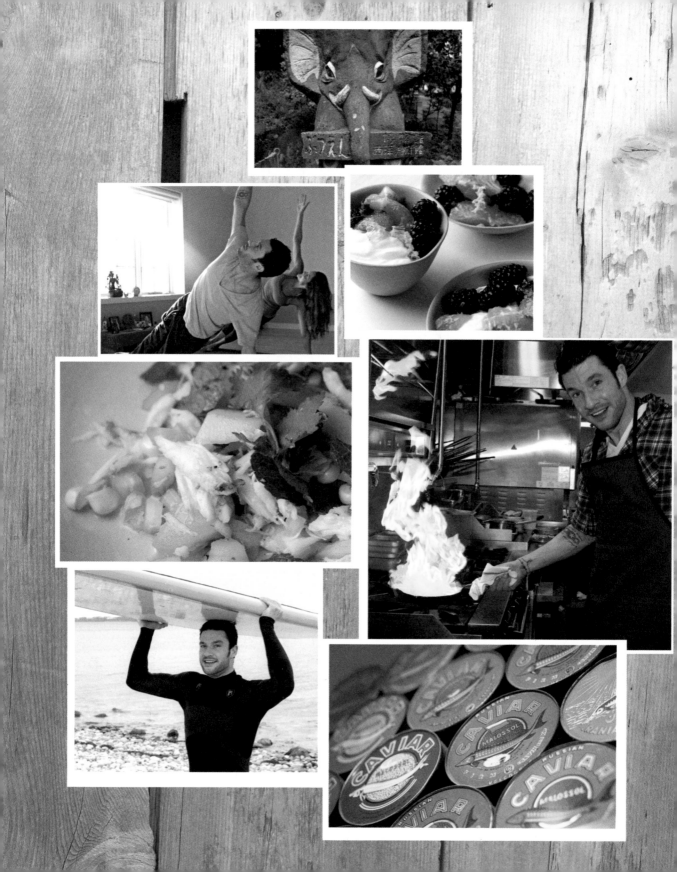

CONTENTS

The *Sweet Life* is a book aimed not only at diabetics but also at anyone who is health conscious, who doesn't want to follow a fad diet but does want to eat great, real food on a regular basis.

PREFACE

I first met Sam while I was a guest judge on *Top Chef* and subsequently had the pleasure of getting to know him better as a frequent guest at his delicious and fun restaurant, the Surf Lodge in Montauk, New York.

If you are reading this, you likely already know that Sam is diabetic and has been since he was a child. When he asked if I would contribute to his book, I was a little curious to see the recipes and dishes he had created for those living with (and without) the disease. As chefs, we like to consider the world wide open to us and never like to work with any constraints as to the ingredients we can use or techniques with which we can cook. I wondered if having to cook with a special diet in mind would limit Sam's creativity. On the contrary, though, I found that Sam was not hemmed in by the limitations; instead he has created a book that is full of recipes that I find clever, inspirational, healthy, and very, very good.

In Sam's cooking both at Surf Lodge and at his newest restaurant, Imperial No. 9, he has a large emphasis on fish and, as it is for me at Le Bernardin, sustainability is of the utmost concern. The food in his restaurants as well as what he offers in this book reflects Sam's beliefs and passions when it comes to food sourcing—be it sustainable fish, meat from local farmers, or artisan and organic produce. You can be assured that Sam's heart, like his food, is in the right place.

As chefs, when we are asked in our restaurants to accommodate certain dietary requirements due to food allergies, intolerances, or other restrictions, we strive to do so while still giving the customer the best food experience we can. This is what Sam Talbot has endeavored to do and has achieved with *The Sweet Life*.

The Sweet Life is a book aimed not only at diabetics but also at anyone who is health conscious, who doesn't want to follow a fad diet but does want to eat great, real food on a regular basis. Beyond the recipes, which feature beautiful, natural ingredients, Sam offers solid advice and sound wisdom for good, healthy living.

This book is destined to become the one in your collection that is dog-eared, stained, and showing the signs of frequent use. *Santé!*

Eric Ripert
Executive Chef/Co-Owner, Le Bernardin

FOREWORD

Managing diabetes is a marathon: a daily challenge to keep blood sugar under control.

Study after study shows that good diabetes control diminishes the risk for eye, nerve, and kidney damage related to diabetes, and the same goes for prevention of heart attacks and strokes. For some people medication may be necessary, but for anyone who has been diagnosed with type 1 or type 2 diabetes or a prediabetic condition, a good diet is essential for keeping blood sugar in check.

From my very first consultation as Sam's endocrinologist, I could tell that his devotion to good diabetes care was matched by a passion for culinary excellence. As both a type 1 diabetic and a healthcare provider, I am always searching for new ways to improve diabetes care both for myself and for my patients and am all too aware of how limited the culinary choices available to those of us on restricted diets can be. In *The Sweet Life,* Sam has used his experiences as a world-renowned chef to show that it is entirely possible to find both health *and* happiness in the kitchen.

Such a resource, sadly, is long overdue, and the need has never been greater. In recent years, diabetes has become a global epidemic; it now afflicts an estimated 285 million people worldwide and is expected to afflict nearly 438 million by the year 2030. Early and aggressive treatment is essential and a healthy diet remains a vital component of successful treatment.

Historically the diabetic diet has been anything but sweet. Doctors denied diabetics many foods rather than empowering them to make healthy, personalized, and well-balanced decisions regarding what to eat and when. Patients were told to follow unrealistically rigid and standardized programs that often left them feeling frustrated, ashamed, and alienated: frustrated with healthcare providers for taking away the basic pleasures of taste, variety, and free will; ashamed when they were unable to follow their doctors' strict instructions, often resulting in a sense of failure and embarrassment during healthcare visits; and alienated from family and friends for not being able to partake in holiday feasts or enjoy the majority of foods served at dinner parties. Variety was "exchanged" for uniformity. Anything sweet was frowned upon.

Fortunately, attitudes toward diabetes and diet are evolving. I always tell my patients that each diabetic needs to follow his or her own cookbook. Each of us has a different metabolism and lifestyle, and different foods affect each of us differently. Diabetics need to be given food options, not orders, and that is precisely what *The Sweet Life* provides. While there may be no perfect recipe for good diabetes control, Sam's approach includes all the right ingredients. Life is meant to be lived and to be enjoyed. Diabetes does not have to take the fun out of food. In the pages that follow, Sam has used his extraordinary talents in the kitchen to reinvent the diabetic diet to include variety, balance, and flavor. As an endocrinologist and type 1 diabetic, I am as excited to recommend the recipes in Sam's new book as I am to try them myself. The days of the boring diabetic diet are over. Bring on variety. Bring on flavor. Bring on *The Sweet Life*!

Dr. Jason C. Baker

Dr. Baker is an endocrinologist and assistant professor of medicine at Weill Cornell Medical College. He is also the founder of Marjorie's Kids, an initiative to improve type 1 diabetes care in the developing world.

. . . it is entirely possible to find both health and happiness in the kitchen.

. . . I learned, at age 12, I had a chronic and
very serious disease I would have
to live with for the rest of my life.

INTRODUCTION

The doctor was "running a little late," the nurse told my mother and me. She said she'd just pop in to his office down the hall to see how long we might have to wait. With the office door ajar, we could hear every word of their conversation. "Does the kid know that he has diabetes yet?" the doctor asked the nurse. That was how I learned, at age 12, I had a chronic and very serious disease I would have to live with for the rest of my life.

Not that I entirely understood what that meant. An uncle had the disease, so I was familiar with diabetes, but age 12 is age 12, and absorbing the full impact of "chronic" or "lifetime" doesn't come easy—if at all. What I did understand was that my mother couldn't hold back her tears the whole time the doctor was talking to us.

"Don't worry, Mom," I said, rising to the occasion as only a 12-year-old can. "We will do just what they tell us to do, and it will be okay." And although I can't honestly say that I have always done exactly what doctors tell me to do all the time, mostly it *has* been okay. In fact, it's been a whole lot better than okay; my life is sweet, and I firmly believe that it can be for all diabetics once you're armed with some helpful information and, of course, a repertoire of really great recipes. And that's where I come in.

That day, my mother dried her tears and announced we were going to Friendly's, where I proceeded to down a half dozen ice cream sundaes, one favorite combination of flavors after another, because, as my Mom said, "this is the last time you can do this."

After that day, the door to that particular kind of sweetness—the hot-fudge-whipped-cream-every-flavor-of-ice-cream-imaginable kind—pretty much slammed shut. But, as the saying goes, another door opened. Lots of other doors. (Just take a look at the dessert recipes in this book!)

Meanwhile, I'm going through as many of those doors as I can as fast as I can. I hope you will come along with me.

DIABETES—AND FOOD

Diabetes is a disease that has been widely known since ancient times. There is as yet no cure. Before the discovery of insulin in the early 1920s, doctors tended to prescribe very restrictive diets—sometimes restrictive to the point of near-starvation—but patients still suffered a range of complications, and most died young.

Today, people with diabetes, whether type 1, like me, or type 2, like 25 million people in this country, can live long, long lives if we are smart about our health and especially about what we eat. Fortunately, we can still eat wonderfully well—so wonderfully well, in fact, that no diabetic ever has to feel that his or her eating is restricted. The recipes in this book will prove my approach to cooking to manage diabetes is as rich as the earth's bounty and as varied as the world's diverse cuisines. It may introduce you to foods you haven't tried before and to methods of preparing "traditional" foods that surprise you. I hope so.

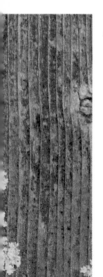

Total Prevalence of Diabetes

Total: 25.8 million children and adults in the United States—8.3 percent of the population—have diabetes.
Diagnosed: 18.8 million people
Undiagnosed: 7.0 million people
Prediabetes: 79 million people
New cases: 1.9 million new cases of diabetes are diagnosed in people aged 20 years and older in 2010.

Data from the 2011 National Diabetes Fact Sheet (released Jan. 26, 2011)

And for you nondiabetics out there, here's a bonus: Eat like a diabetic, using the recipes in this book, and you'll be embracing a food philosophy that doctors and nutritionists recommend to keep you healthy for a lifetime. In fact, if everybody ate like a diabetic, we could make a major dent in the nation's rates of obesity, heart disease, and a range of other debilitating ailments linked to diet. Follow the recipes in this book, and you'll be getting healthy on haute cuisine. Not a bad deal.

At the heart of eating like a diabetic is paying attention—to what you eat, when, how much—and that's probably a good idea for everyone. For all diabetics, it's the front line of dealing with the disease, the first step in controlling blood sugar levels. The reason this is so critical all comes back to one thing: insulin.

Insulin is a hormone produced by the pancreas. Its function is to move sugar out of the bloodstream into the various cells of your body to power up your muscles and tissues. In healthy folks, it's a simple process: Your body breaks down carbohydrates in food—and this can be any food that contains carbs, whether it's a bowl of mashed potatoes, a glass of soda, or a chocolate brownie—into glucose (sugars). The sugars enter the bloodstream and the insulin helps move them out of the bloodstream and into the various cells of the body. If insulin isn't present (or isn't working well), the blood sugar is unable to get into the cells of the body and it builds up in the bloodstream. High blood sugar, which can lead to insufficient energy for the body and slow blood circulation, is bad for the functioning of the body's cells and blood. Left untreated, it can lead to very serious complications. Bad all around.

With type 1 diabetes, the so-called childhood diabetes that I have, the body just stops producing insulin. So in addition to paying attention to what we eat, we have to provide our bodies with insulin through a needle or a pen or pump it via a catheter under the skin. In type 2 diabetes, also called adult onset diabetes, the pancreas still produces insulin, but the hormone doesn't work very efficiently or effectively. For the most part, people with type 2 diabetes can control the disease through eating a modified diet, getting more exercise, losing weight, and in some cases taking meds.

Whether you are currently taking supplemental insulin or managing your condition through diet, you should always pay attention to the food you eat. I can't truthfully say I always eat only the foods I should, but on those occasions when I do throw caution to the wind, I do so mindfully, and I know how to deal with any consequences. And it's only through years of learning how my body responds to different foods and how I can mitigate those responses effectively and safely that I can break the rules now and again. It's a process of discovery that didn't happen overnight.

A CHEF'S EDUCATION

I got my first cooking job when I was 15, just a few years after my diabetes diagnosis. I had fallen in love with food at my grandparents' house in Ohio, where I first tasted scrambled eggs with Cheddar cheese, the eggs fresh from a local farm just 30 miles away. Once you've had fresh eggs, nothing else will do. Thus began my love affair with all things edible.

But it was the cooking job that made me get serious about both food and diabetes. I cooked all through high school and college, using my body as a laboratory for educating myself about food and my disease. It's funny: I absolutely suck at math, but I can calculate carbohydrates in my head at record speed. Over the years I've experimented endlessly with particular foods and amounts of foods and observed their effect on my insulin levels and blood sugar levels.

Along the way I learned a lot about my body, my disease, and the benefits of eating fresh, unprocessed foods, both as a diabetic and as a chef. Using only unadulterated, natural foods allowed me to know exactly what I was eating at any given time; food that had never seen the inside of a packaging plant couldn't be harboring any hidden sugars, starches, or other additives that might do a number on my blood sugar without my knowing it. It also, quite simply, just tasted better. That helped me to understand the importance of supporting local food products and the many advantages of sustainability in all its forms. (It turns out that the food that sustains me best is also the food that helps sustain the delicate ecosystem we depend on for sustenance.) I came to insist on using food that I could trace to accountable suppliers, and to cherish artisanal food products. These were reasoned conclusions based on the empirical evidence of what worked for my health and at the same time made for really great cuisine. That philosophy is present in every recipe in this book.

But I still obsess. Most people clock in from 9 to 5 and probably don't think about food except when they sit down to eat. Me, I work with food all day and all evening, then go home and think about food through the night, often dream about it, and wake up thinking

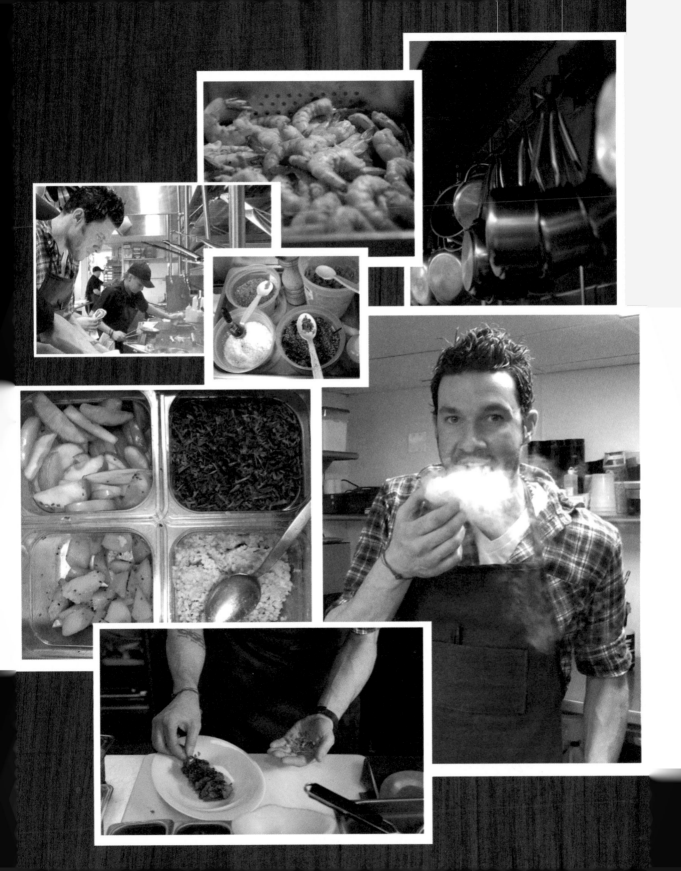

about it some more. It's how I'm wired. As a diabetic and a chef, I have to be. Food reaches into every part of my life, and frankly, I can't separate being a diabetic from being a chef. My love for cooking has made me a healthier diabetic, and being a diabetic has made me a better cook. It definitely informs the food I serve to customers at my restaurants, Imperial No. 9 in New York City and The Surf Lodge out on Long Island, though you'd never mistake the food on those menus as "health food" or in any way austere.

Anyone concerned about avoiding diabetes would do well to eat the way we do and follow the recipes in this book. And given the way far too many Americans eat these days, just about everyone is vulnerable to this disease. The one thing they don't tell you when you get those first lectures on carbs in your body is that you're about to become a model of smart eating for people who don't even have the disease. But it's true. If everyone ate the way diabetics should eat, the way these recipes tell us to eat, we'd all be healthy and we'd all eat well. How sweet is that?

Bottom line: If you or someone you love is living with diabetes, you owe it to yourself to learn as much as you can about food, and how it can have an enormous impact on everyone's health (not to mention the health of the planet!).

PARAMETERS

Believe it or not, there are actually one or two bonuses to having diabetes—a couple of perks we get that others don't. At school, I was allowed to eat a Snickers bar in class, to the envy of all the other kids, and there have been times at work when I just had to walk off the job and head for home because I knew I was going to crash. And yes, I admit it, I've used the excuse to get out of a boring social studies class at school or cruise to the front of a long security line at the airport because I "had to" get to some juice fast. (My friend Willie Garson, of *Sex and the City* fame, claims these special privileges have spawned a phenomenon he has dubbed the "wannabetic"—the totally undiabetic individual who carries syringes and a nearly empty bottle of insulin in order to cop some of these same advantages. I think he's kidding. . . .)

Other than those rare bonuses, however, I can't say I'm grateful to have diabetes. No one wants to live with a dangerous disease. But living with the disease—and therefore being forced to live within certain parameters—has taught me some valuable lessons.

Kids and Diabetes

One great perk of being a chef (and getting some media attention from my stint on *Top Chef*) is being able to bring attention to causes I believe in, which is why I've teamed up with the JDRF (Juvenile Diabetes Research Foundation), an organization that provides resources for diabetics and is working for better ways to create and ultimately cure type 1 diabetes. It's a great resource for anyone with the disease, especially kids. I know what they're going through, and I know what their concerned parents are going through, too. I've seen it in action—my own mother following me around with a meter and finger pricker to make sure I was checking my blood sugar. Or the school nurse, Miss Carosella—bless her—running down the hallway in front of me yelling at me to hurry up, run faster, because my blood sugar had just hit 300 and we had to act fast! I remember the times I had to run off the field in

football practice and grab—quick!—a bottle of juice. Or trying to explain to my high school sweetheart exactly why there were some things in life I couldn't do, some other things I had to do, and how my life was just—well, different.

Not easy when you're a kid. Not easy at all.

I can't go through it for the kids out there who have been diagnosed with diabetes, or for the men and women in college or in their twenties or even thirties still trying to adjust to a life that just isn't what they expected. I can only say that I too was terrified, I too was discombobulated, and I too was totally uncertain about everything. But now I'm not.

Believe me when I tell you that the uncertain becomes stable, and the discombobulated falls into place, and the terrifying recedes. And one day you wake up and realize that you're in control. Your disease is not your destiny. It doesn't own you; you own it. Once you've got that nailed, you're really living large.

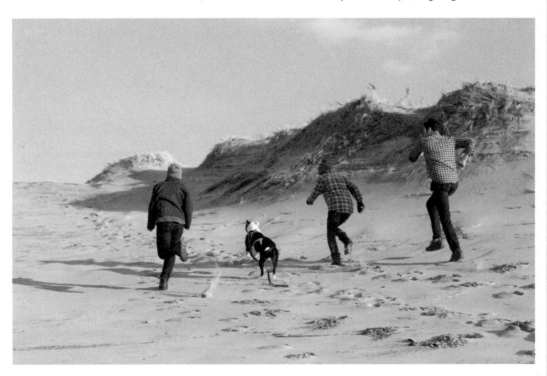

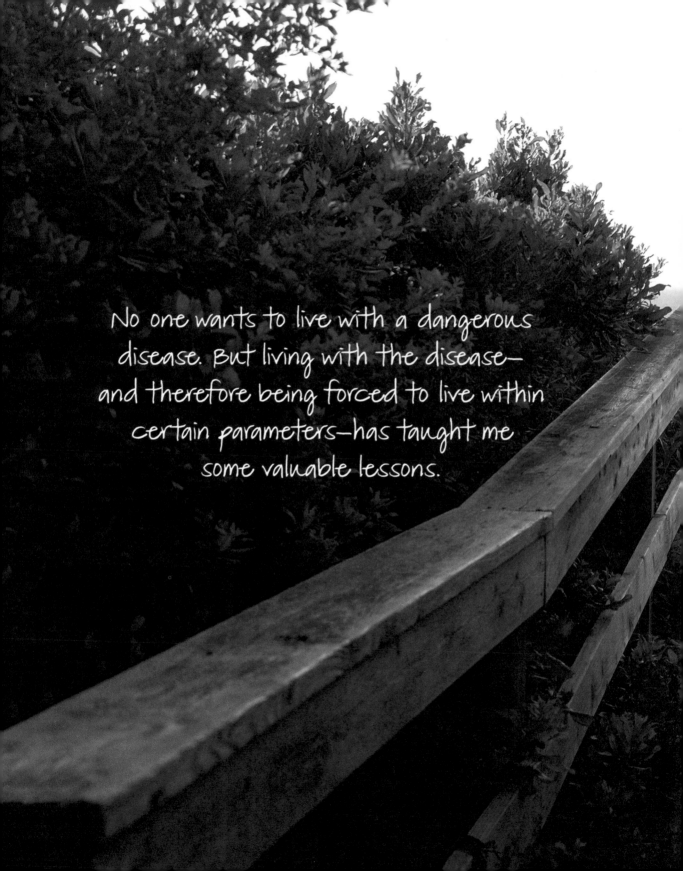

No one wants to live with a dangerous disease. But living with the disease— and therefore being forced to live within certain parameters—has taught me some valuable lessons.

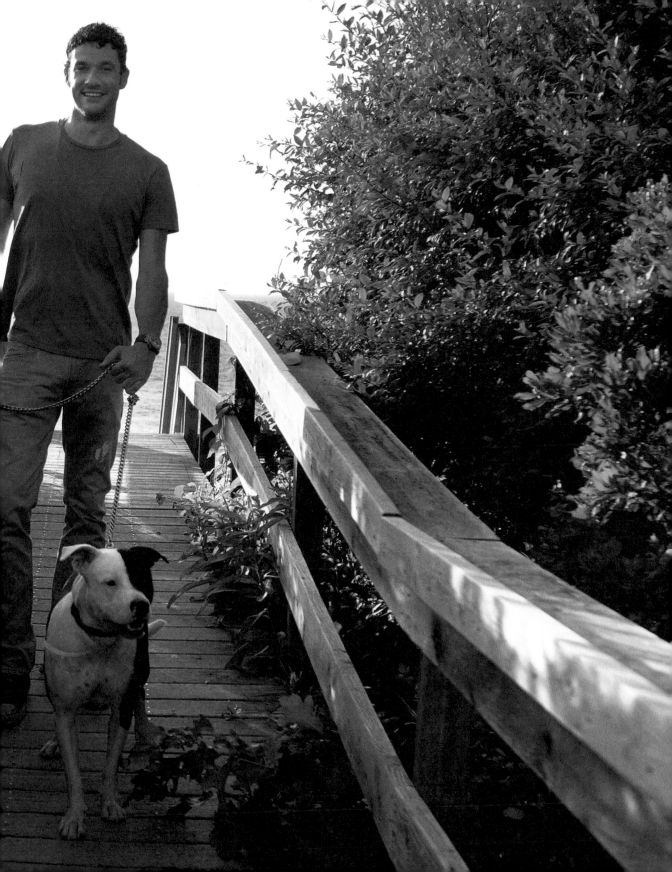

First, it has made it imperative for me to know about food—what it is, what it does, where it comes from, how it gets to us. Diabetics have to know this because the cause-and-effect response to what we put into our bodies is so immediate and so profound. That's why I'm so adamant about knowing the source of the food I prepare, how it was grown or killed, whether other species were harmed in the process, how long and in what conditions it traveled to get to me, and how it was handled and by whom. I know if I start with exacting standards and obtain the highest quality product, I'm more than halfway to preparing superb meals for my restaurant guests and for myself at home.

Second, I think diabetes has given me the gift of focus; it forces me to live in a thoughtful way. Every day, those of us who have this disease have to focus on what's ahead, figure out the shape of our day, plan when and where and what we will eat during the day to keep our blood sugar level in its healthy range. Or to be ready to act on the spot if and when our level takes a dive or spikes upward.

We can't overdo things, but we also can't under-do things. Overdo or under-do, and we risk our blood sugar going awry. And when our blood sugar goes awry, so does everything else: our mood, good sense, emotions, even our productivity.

PLEASE PLAY WITH YOUR FOOD!

Lots of people are taught not to play with food. I play with it, touch it, take it apart and put it back together, research it, film it, blog about it, paint images of it on huge canvases—and make my living cooking it. The aim is always to find a better way to bring out the best in a high-quality product, and to do so without adding a bunch of unnecessary ingredients that can have an unwanted effect on my blood sugar levels. I never want to obscure the taste or texture of an ingredient; I want to help it emerge.

Ironically, that's pretty much why I lost on *Top Chef*. It was the penultimate episode. I was on track to win the thing, or so many people (including me!) thought. I had dominated the quickfire challenges, winning several back to back and had done very well across the board; I was even voted Fan Favorite. But on this episode, the judges were torn between my entry and Ilan's, conceding that they couldn't find anything bad to say about either one of our dishes. So judge Tom Colicchio seized on a technicality. "Well," he said, "Sam didn't cook anything in this challenge."

Didn't cook anything? It was a ceviche—a beautiful piece of raw opakapaka, the famous Hawaiian pink snapper, marinated in yuzu, a tart and aromatic citrus juice, and rice vinegar. In a ceviche, the marinade itself "cooks" the fish; the various ingredients react with one another to transform the fish and give the dish its particular texture and taste. (Technically speaking, the citric acid denatures the protein in the fish—not unlike a pickling process.) True, no heat was applied, and if "applying heat" is your definition of cooking, then I guess you could say my ceviche wasn't "cooked." In any event, I was eliminated from the competition.

Go figure.

Top Chef was a valuable experience, and I learned a lot from it, but I'll stick to my own definition of cooking and my own ideas about winning food. For me, winning food is healthy, obtained in a sustainable way, and inspired by a real passion for food and cooking. That's true for every single recipe in this book.

Inspiration is the one ingredient every chef needs, whether you're creating a dessert of grilled peaches with mascarpone, lemon, and vincotto for diners in a stylish Manhattan restaurant or whipping up some scrambled eggs on a Sunday morning and wondering what it would taste like if you tossed in—what? A drop of Tabasco sauce? A bit of aged Cheddar? Some of that leftover squash? A crushed basil leaf? It doesn't matter where or when or how the inspiration happens, so long as it happens. Boom! It knocks you right out. Then it's go time, and nothing is better, nothing is as good. When it happens to me, I feel stoked, the adrenaline starts flowing, and I feel like I'm on cloud nine.

Inspiration isn't selfish; it has to be shared. Being executive chef of a restaurant is the perfect opportunity for sharing. I traveled to Japan when I was in the midst of starting up Imperial No. 9 and learned a bunch of new things about Japanese cuisine. What I learned fired me up. I brought that inspiration home and made it a part of some very thoughtful dishes on the menu at the restaurant, and now it is a great feeling to see guests literally tasting my inspiration.

You can't put a price tag on that. It is so worth the work that inspiration sets in motion—and it sets in motion an immense amount of work. But it feels awfully good to do work you love. When that switch goes off and you're in the groove of inspiration, then you can be pretty confident that everything you do will be at its best.

Healthy and delicious eating. Food that is simple, pared down to fresh, real, sustainably produced ingredients. No show business, no gimmicks, no "butter-poached spot prawns with celeriac-laced truffle fries and maple-bacon-scented Brussels sprouts topped with crunchy croutons and basil." My brain hurts from tapping this out on the keyboard, let alone eating it.

Food that mixes and matches all the diverse tastes of many cultures, ideas, sources of inspiration.

Food that delights the palate while it strengthens the body, fuels the muscles and tissues, and nurtures the organs that keep us going and keep us healthy.

What's good for us is good for the planet and good to taste: This is what inspires me, and being diabetic is what got me here.

I hope the recipes in this book convince you of that at least when it comes to eating. The recipes offer irrefutable evidence there is no flavor on this earth we diabetics have to miss out on. We can and should experience the whole fantastically diverse bounty of eating that the world has to offer. We can and should play with this bounty. We're not surrendering anything when it comes to eating; on the contrary, we're taking charge of our lives and eating the best and most delicious foods that earth and ocean have to offer—limited only by our own creativity—because the best and most delicious are the healthiest as well.

To me, that's inspiring, and as I hope you've gathered by now, inspiration is my drug of choice.

I've written this book to share some of my favorite ways to transform blood-sugar friendly foods—those low on the glycemic index but high on the flavor scale—into beautiful, mind-blowingly delicious foods like those I eat every day and serve to friends (and customers) all year round.

I hope they will help you manage your diabetes or prediabetic condition; I know they will make your life more sweet.

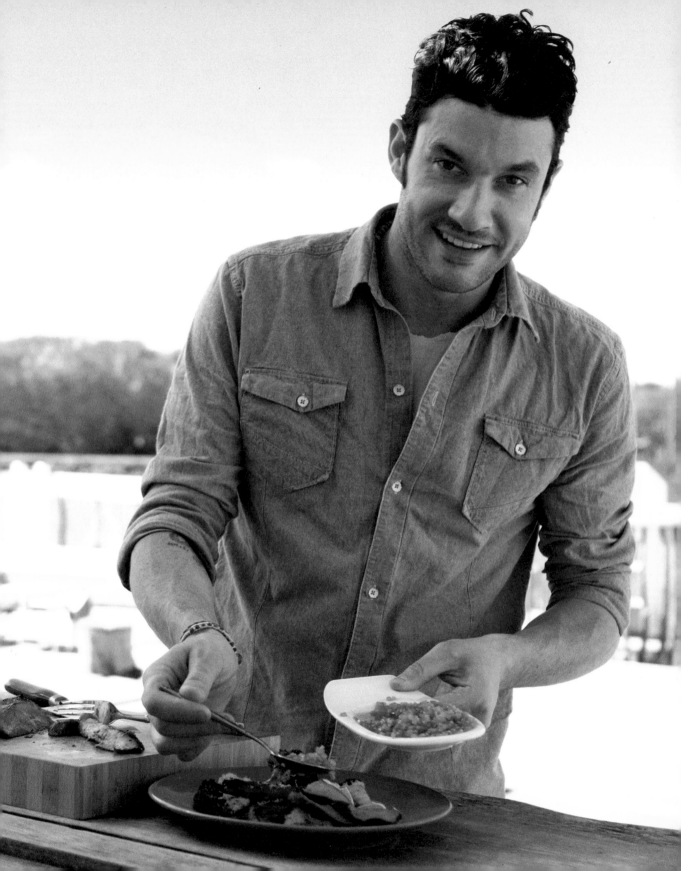

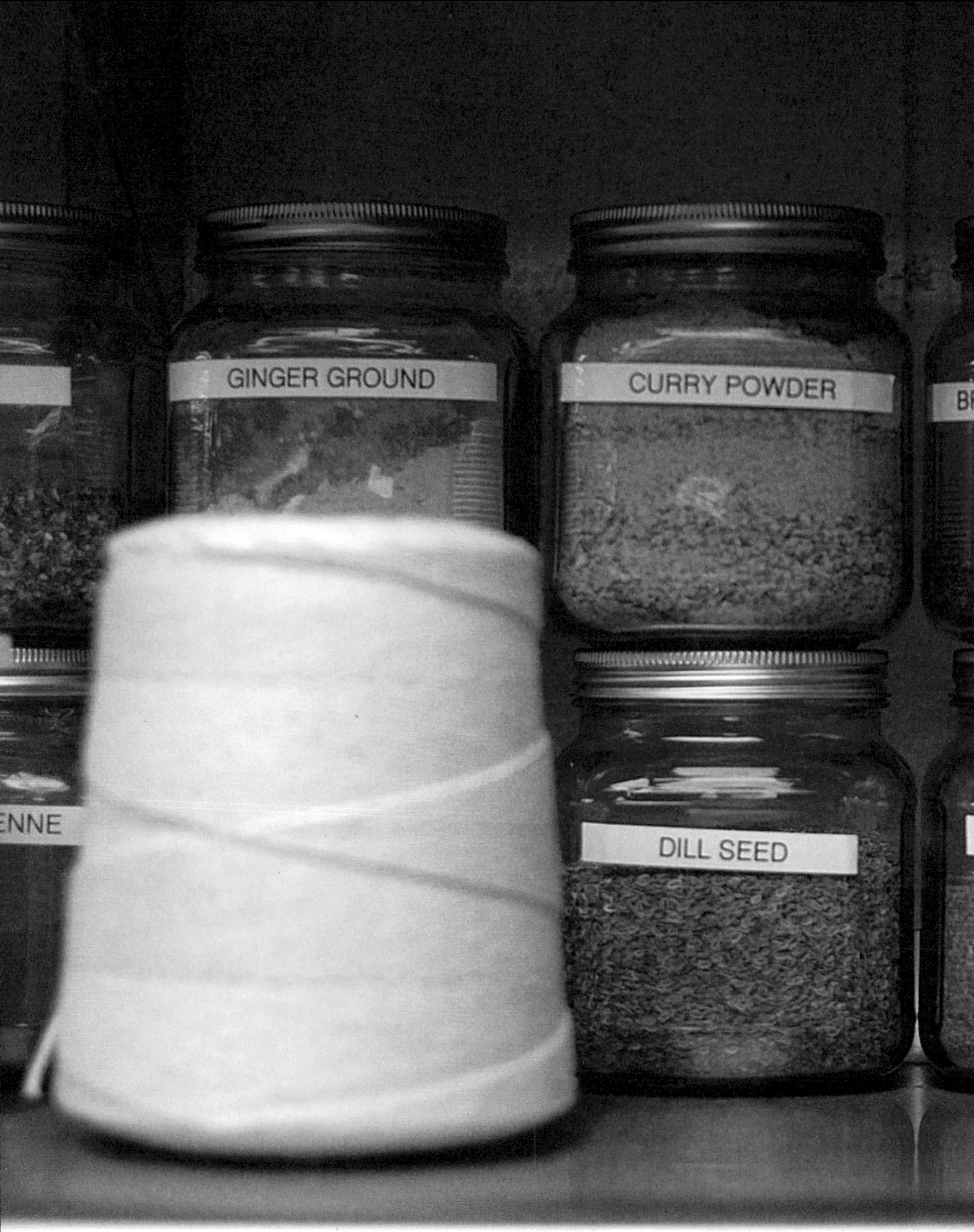
GINGER GROUND
CURRY POWDER
DILL SEED

Chapter One

WELCOME
TO MY
KITCHEN*

*Notice I didn't say *Diabetic* Kitchen?

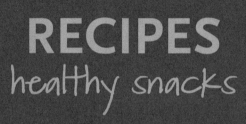

RECIPES
healthy snacks

've been eating and cooking with one eye on the stove and the other on my blood sugar levels for just about as long as I can remember. Maybe you're a little newer to all this, or maybe you're ready for a change from the tried and true recipes (or worse, prefab "diabetic" products off the shelf) you've come to rely on to keep things on an even keel. Are you cooking for someone you care about who has been told that unless they change their eating habits, their prediabetic condition can develop into full-blown diabetes? Whatever your reason for picking up this book, you're going to be making food that I have been passionate about for many years and many more to come, so please cook nice.

Let me get one thing out of the way right off the bat: As far as I'm concerned there is nothing that is completely off limits for people with diabetes, period, end of story. When I first got my diagnosis the nurse handed my mother a list of forbidden foods—soda, cookies and crackers, fried foods, ice cream, French fries, breakfast cereal—pretty much everything on an 11-year-old's top 10 list. But if you really think about it, none of these is a food that anyone, regardless of health status, should be chowing down on regularly. If I get together with some friends back home for a fish fry, or have a bit of birthday cake at a friend's party, I do so knowing it's likely to have an effect on my blood sugar, and I deal with it. And eat better for the rest of the day.

While nothing is completely off the menu, you do have to put a little thought into putting that menu together every day. For diabetics, eating well is less a matter of avoiding foods that rate high on the glycemic index than it is of keeping track of the total grams of carbs you take in at any given meal and throughout the course of the day. Take beets, for example. They are one of my very favorite vegetables and are packed with the kinds of vitamins and minerals a potato would kill for. Sure they are relatively high in carbs, but they're also delicious and earthy and nutritious. I just don't eat them at every meal and I wouldn't pair them with another high-carb food like rice. Keep in mind too that food affects everyone differently, and you may just need to experiment to see which foods affect your blood glucose in a big way.

In general I try not to exceed 25 to 30 grams of carbs per meal, 80 to 90 per day; you and your doctor should decide what's appropriate for you. That said, after 20 years, I can make calculations like these in my head, and between frequent testing of my blood glucose throughout the day, and balancing the carbs I take in with a greater proportion of low-carb veggies, protein, and fats, I don't get too many unhappy surprises.

FUELING UP

Even with insulin supplying what our bodies lack, we diabetics are always walking a fine line between getting some nutrients in us and making sure they're the kind of nutrients that will keep our blood sugar at the right level. Taste has usually come in a poor third after those two goals are met.

Often, the key is not only *what* we eat but *when* we eat, and that's a challenge I face just about every day. After all, night is the busiest part of a chef's workday. Just as the guests sit down to a pleasant and relaxing dinner, my workplace—the restaurant kitchen—is at its absolute peak of activity. We are all rushed off our feet and up to our necks with work.

That sort of nonstop activity—with no chance to break for a bite of something healthy, much less to sit down for a real meal—is a no-no for diabetics. Actually, it's a no-no for everybody, but worse for us. We're supposed to eat at regular intervals, and I can assure you that there is no such thing as a regular interval in a New York City restaurant kitchen. I'm lucky in that I can almost always find some good, healthy food to answer the call. I try to have a light lunch at around 11:00 in the morning and rustle up some sort of supper for myself around 5:00 p.m., *before* the restaurant kitchen tips over into chaos. Then as things calm down a bit around 10:30 or so, I have a light, low-carb, low-fat, very clean snack just to maintain my blood sugar level—something sautéed like broccoli rabe. You'll need to work out a schedule that fits with your daily routine. Just remember that a crazy busy day is no excuse for letting your blood sugar level go.

SQUIRREL FOOD

Which brings me to the healthy snacks you'll find in this chapter. When you're *out there*, on the move, doing what you do to win the world, food that isn't fast and easy won't cut it. Leisurely meals are for weekends, special occasions, first dates, special dates, very special dates. The rest of the time, it's snacks, lunches, and whatever you can grab. Of course, for diabetics—and for those of you trying to eat healthy the way we diabetics have to—a snack or even the smallest fistful of whatever you have time to munch on must still offer a nutritional benefit, one that won't wreak havoc with blood sugar. And if you're me, it also has to taste totally awesome, or what's the point?

You'll notice a number of these snack recipes contain nuts and seeds—well, nuts *are* seeds actually; that is, they contain the seed as well as the fruit of their plant. There's a good reason I use them in so many recipes here: They have a high oil content, which makes them an exceptional source of energy. In fact, that's pretty much why squirrels spend the entire fall season gathering acorns and—wait for it—squirreling them away. The nuts will keep them alive and well fed as they work through the autumn, the entire winter, and well into early spring—so long as their stashes aren't found and stolen by bears or other lazier but bigger species who would just as soon let the squirrels do the work while they reap the results.

You probably won't have that problem, which is good, because what works for squirrels works also for us humans. Nuts and seeds are energy powerhouses. Try this: Maybe sometime around the middle of the afternoon, when you feel your vigor is flagging a bit, grab a Coconut Açai Granola Crumble (page 23), or maybe some Toasted Hemp Seeds with Golden Berry and Cocoa (page 24), and the odds are better than good that you'll soon feel a new burst of strength and vitality. Honest.

And the good part—especially for diabetics or prediabetics—is that nuts and seeds are very low on the glycemic index, which makes them particularly good for people with insulin resistance problems. Any way you crack them, nuts and seeds are high-energy foods that help keep blood sugar levels under control. And these delicious snacks will keep you going all day—even if your day keeps you away from home till late at night.

Right on Target

Blood glucose levels fluctuate throughout the day, not just before you eat, but after as well. If you are unsure how your body reacts to a particular food you may need to monitor your blood glucose a few times to get a real fix on it, usually once before you eat, and then 1, 2, or 3 hours after you've eaten.

Generally you're looking for results in this range:

Before meals: 90–130 mg/dl
1 hour after eating:
less than 180 mg/dl
2 hours after eating:
less than 160 mg/dl
3 hours after eating:
less than 140 mg/dl

If your postmeal levels are clocking in a good deal higher than this, you probably need to make some adjustments to the menu, either by controlling portion size or replacing some high-carb components with ingredients that are kinder to your body.

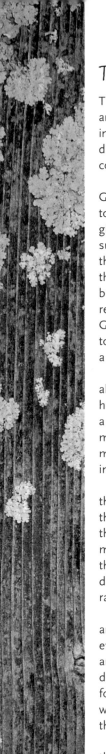

The Lowdown on High GI

There's been a lot of talk about glycemic index and glycemic load recently, and both are important to understand—and not just for diabetics. Fortunately, the terms are a lot less complicated than they sound.

"Glycemic" comes from the same ancient Greek root as "glucose," so you know it has to do with sugar. Indeed it does: The glycemic index ranks a food's effect on blood sugar level; the higher the ranking, the faster the food's glucose content is broken down by the digestive process and sent into the bloodstream. Glucose itself is the point of reference; it has a glycemic-index ranking, or GI, of 100. So other foods are ranked relative to that standard. Almonds, for example, have a GI of 15; hemp seed is ranked at 35.

Obviously, for diabetics, prediabetics, and all of you out there who are trying to eat healthy to avoid diabetes forever, foods with a lower glycemic-index rating are better. It means that the carbs in the food break down more slowly and that the glucose is absorbed into the bloodstream more gradually.

The only problem with measuring GI is that it doesn't take into account how much of the food you're actually eating, so to cover that failure, scientists developed the glycemic load (GL) measurement. GL multiplies the GI of a food by the amount of carbohydrate it contains, then divides by 100, so its ranking combines both quantity and quality.

This makes sense, because a very small amount of a high-GI food may have no worse effect on blood sugar level than a very large amount of a low-GI food. So certainly for diabetics, GL is more useful measurement for avoiding sudden spikes in blood sugar—which are what's really bad for us—and therefore for managing our levels.

Here is a list of some common foods and their GI value to give you a sense of it. (Note that nonstarchy vegetables are rarely included in these studies because they have such minimal glycemic impact; for information on some common fruits, see page 216.)

FOOD	GI	GL
Snacks		
Hummus	67	0 (about 1 ounce)
Peanuts	14	1 (about 2 ounces)
Cashews	22	3 (about 2 ounces)
Milk chocolate	43	12 (1 bar)
Potato chips	54	11 (about 2 ounces)
Corn chips	63	17 (about 2 ounces)
Popcorn	72	8 (about 2 cups, popped)
Jelly beans	78	22 (about 1 ounce)
Pretzels	83	16 (about 1 ounce)
Breads		
Pumpernickel bread	41	5 (1 slice)
Sourdough bread	54	8 (1 slice)
Stone ground whole wheat bread	52	6 (1 slice)
Pita, whole wheat	57	10 (1 4" pita)
Whole meal rye	58	8 (1 slice)
Croissant	67	17 (1 medium)
Taco shell	68	8 (1 6½" shell)
Vegetables		
Tomatoes	15	2 (1 medium)
Beets	64	5 (about ½ cup)
Parsnips	97	12 (about ½ cup)
Instant potatoes	85	17 (¾ cup)
Pumpkin	75	9 (about ½ cup)
Carrots	47	3 (about ½ cup)
Peas	48	3 (½ cup)

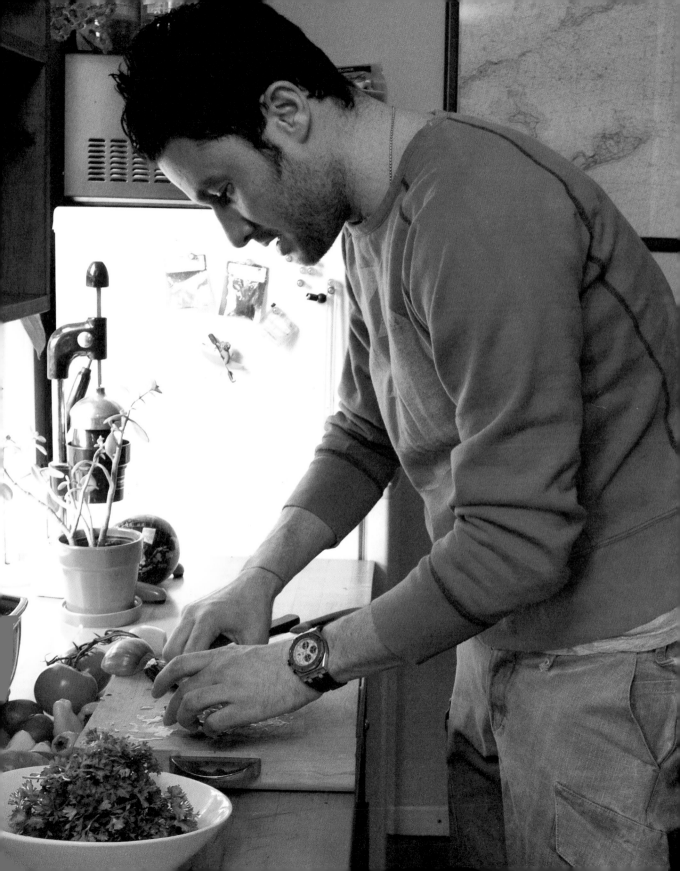

Coconut Açai Granola Crumble

I have always loved granola—since I was a young kid. The problem was that most of the store-bought brands of granola cereals and granola bars were always high in carbs and sugar. And while there is some good stuff out there now, mine quite simply is better. Sprinkle a small handful into a bowl of almond milk or over a cup of yogurt for a really good snack.

Preheat the oven to 300°F. Line a baking sheet with parchment paper.

In a large bowl, combine the oats, oat flour, coconut, sesame seeds, bran flakes, almonds, hazelnuts, pecans, and pistachios. Then gently mix in the cacao nibs, goji berries, golden berries, mulberries, açai powder, sweetener, oil, and agave nectar.

Spread the mixture evenly on the baking sheet. Bake until the granola is golden brown and fragrant, about 1 hour.

Remove from the oven and set aside to cool to room temperature, 20 to 30 minutes. Once it's cooled, break the granola into pieces and enjoy.

PER SERVING: 290 calories, 7 g protein, 35 g carbohydrates, 14 g total fat (3 g saturated), 0 mg cholesterol, 5 g fiber, 20 mg sodium

- 3 cups old-fashioned rolled oats
- ½ cup oat flour
- ½ cup unsweetened shredded coconut
- ¼ cup sesame seeds
- ¼ cup bran flake cereal
- ¼ cup sliced almonds
- ¼ cup chopped hazelnuts
- ¼ cup chopped pecans
- ¼ cup chopped pistachios
- 2 tablespoons cacao nibs
- 2 tablespoons goji berries
- 2 tablespoons golden berries
- 2 tablespoons dried mulberries
- 1 tablespoon açai powder
- Granulated stevia extract equivalent to ¾ cup sugar
- 2 tablespoons canola oil
- ½ cup agave nectar

Toasted Hemp Seeds with Golden Berry and Cocoa

12

Hemp is the soft fiber cultivated from the cannabis plant, but don't worry, what we're talking about here are the seeds, which contain all the essential amino and fatty acids for life and health. Honestly. They're also unbelievably versatile: Shovel them down raw, grind them into a hemp meal, use them in tea and baking. Here I'm pairing the toasted seeds with golden berry, a tomato-like fruit with amazing anti-inflammatory and anti-oxidant properties for which, like açai, we owe a debt to South America.

In a large skillet, heat the oil over medium-high heat. Add the hemp seeds and toast, tossing frequently, until the seeds are fragrant and golden brown, 4 to 5 minutes.

Transfer the toasted hemp seeds to a medium bowl and add the golden berries, cocoa nibs, salt, and pepper. Set out for people to enjoy.

- 1 tablespoon olive oil
- 2 cups hemp seeds
- ½ cup golden berries
- ½ cup cocoa nibs
- 1 teaspoon fine sea salt
- ½ teaspoon freshly ground black pepper

PER SERVING: 191 calories, 9 g protein, 7 g carbohydrates, 6 g total fat (2 g saturated), 0 mg cholesterol, 2 g fiber, 136 mg sodium

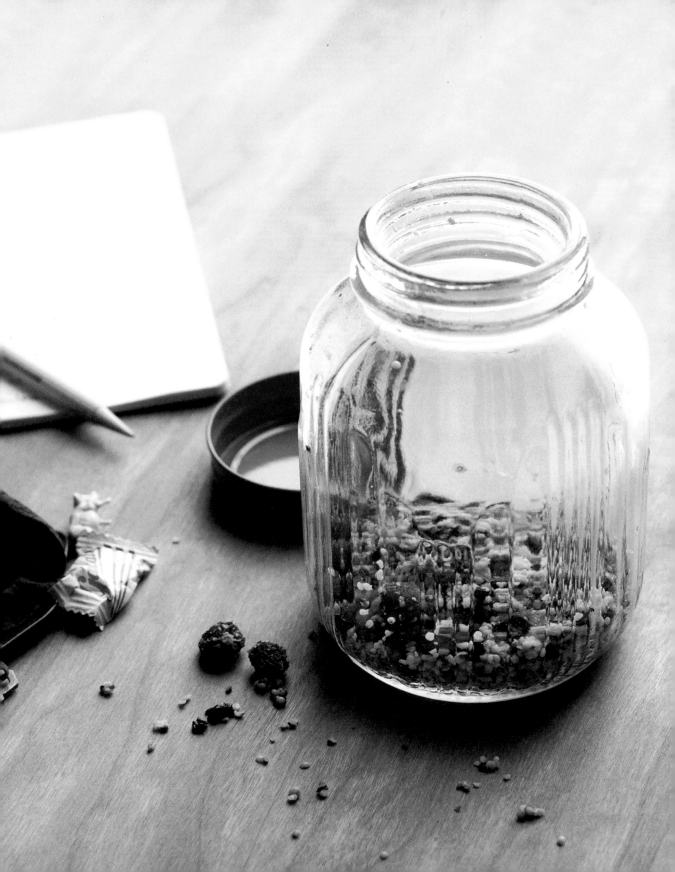

Roasted Seed Trail Mix

Don't leave home without trail mix. You want a healthful snack with you whenever you hit the road—whether the road is a path in the Rockies or Main Street, Yourtown. For one thing, you can't be sure the food you'll find available when the munchies attack is going to be anything but junk. For another thing, when you need a quick hit, you don't want that hit to be a high-priced meal at the nearest restaurant. Prepared in advance, this trail mix balances just the right ratio of carbohydrates to protein to fat. Accompany it with a low-calorie beverage, and it can be a full meal. Make up a bunch, grab as you go . . .

Preheat the oven to 400°F. Line a rimmed baking sheet with parchment paper.

In a large bowl, combine the watermelon seeds, pumpkin seeds, sunflower seeds, soy nuts, almonds, cocoa nibs, cinnamon, salt, and pepper. Drizzle with the oil and vanilla and mix thoroughly.

Spread the mixture on the baking sheet and bake until the seeds are golden brown and toasted, 6 to 8 minutes. You'll smell them when they are ready. Take the baking sheet out of the oven and transfer the trail mix to a bowl for everyone to enjoy. Store any leftovers in an airtight container at room temperature for up to 2 weeks.

PER SERVING: 388 calories, 11 g protein, 15 g carbohydrates, 32 g total fat (6 g saturated), 0 mg cholesterol, 7 g fiber, 470 mg sodium

¼ cup fresh or roasted watermelon seeds

¼ cup raw pumpkin seeds (pepitas)

¼ cup raw sunflower seeds

¼ cup chopped soy nuts

¼ cup almonds

¼ cup sweetened cocoa nibs

1 teaspoon ground cinnamon

1 teaspoon coarse sea salt

½ teaspoon freshly ground black pepper

2 tablespoons extra-virgin olive oil

1 teaspoon pure vanilla extract

Cucumber Kimchi

I love kimchi but don't always have time to track down the special Korean chili powder to make it from scratch—or to allow it to ferment fully. Starting with purchased kimchi, either from the refrigerated case at your supermarket, the health food store, or your farmers' market, makes it super quick and easy to have authentic-tasting kimchi in a fraction of the time. Taste your mixture before adding salt or pepper, as the purchased kimchi may have enough seasoning.

Halve the cucumbers crosswise, then lengthwise, and lengthwise again to make long spears. Place in a mixing bowl and add the kimchi, cabbage, scallions, garlic, ginger, honey, sesame seeds, lime zest and juice, and salt and pepper to taste. Mix gently with a rubber spatula.

Cover the bowl with plastic and refrigerate at least 4 hours (24 hours is better still) before serving. Store leftovers in the refrigerator for up to 4 days.

PER SERVING: 97 calories, 3 g protein, 19 g carbohydrates, 2 g total fat (0 g saturated), 0 mg cholesterol, 4 g fiber, 498 mg sodium

4 **Kirby or 2 hothouse cucumbers**

12 **ounces prepared kimchi**

1 **cup napa cabbage, cut lengthwise in thin strips**

4 **scallions (white and green parts), thinly sliced**

5 **garlic cloves, finely chopped**

3 **tablespoons grated ginger**

3 **tablespoons honey**

2 **tablespoons sesame seeds**

Zest and juice of 1 lime

Salt and freshly ground black pepper, as needed

Kale Chips with Toasted Nori

I love it when America obsesses over something and it really takes off. And today, people are going nuts over kale, which is a good thing because kale is an amazing source of vitamin A. Paired with the toasty, sea-mineral accent of roasted nori—itself a nutritional powerhouse of both vitamin A and calcium—it makes a delicious, super-healthy alternative to the standard football-watching fare. With the right amount of seasoning, these are a knockout.

Preheat the oven to 350°F. Line 2 baking sheets with foil or parchment paper.

In a large bowl, combine the kale, nori, and oil and toss until coated. Spread the kale and nori on the baking sheets and sprinkle with the salt and pepper. Bake until the kale and nori are crispy, 6 to 8 minutes. Be careful not to cook much longer, or the nori and kale will turn dark and bitter.

Remove from the oven and sprinkle with the lemon zest. Let cool to room temperature before serving.

PER SERVING: 183 calories, 4 g protein, 12 g carbohydrates, 15 g total fat (2 g saturated), 0 mg cholesterol, 3 g fiber, 467 mg sodium

- 1 large bunch (about 1¼ pounds) kale, stems and center ribs discarded, leaves roughly torn

- 2 sheets nori, cut into 1 x 2-inch strips

- ¼ cup Roasted Garlic Oil (page 93)

- 1 teaspoon coarse sea salt

- ½ teaspoon freshly ground black pepper

- Grated zest of 1 lemon

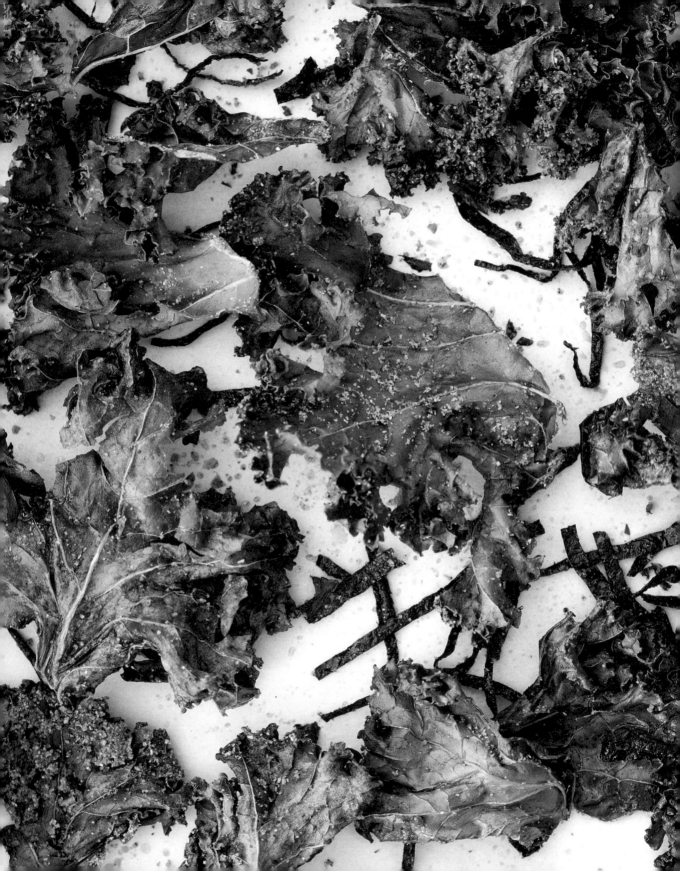

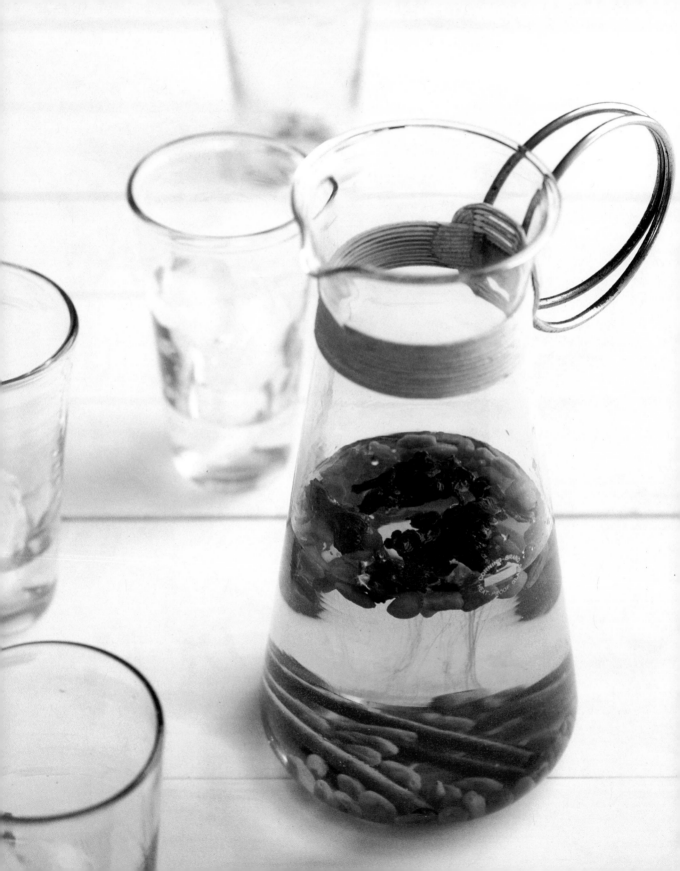

Hibiscus and Goji Iced Tea

When I started making this tea a couple of years ago, I was using only the goji portion of the recipe. Then I hit on the idea of adding the hibiscus. (The best-quality spices and herbs come from San Francisco–based Le Sanctuaire—the best in the business, hands down, and one of my purveyors for the restaurant, where I use hibiscus in a few of the menu items.) Anyway, I took some hibiscus home and added a bit of it to the tea—and it got way better. So I started researching hibiscus and discovered the benefits of having it in your routine. It has all sorts of health and weight loss benefits, so I like how this whole thing worked out.

In a large saucepan, bring 2 quarts of water to a boil over medium-high heat. Remove the pan from the heat and add the goji berries, hibiscus flower, agave nectar, and cinnamon sticks. Let the tea steep for at least 25 minutes, then whisk the mixture vigorously for about 30 seconds to combine the flavors.

Fill a tall glass three-quarters full with ice. Strain the tea through a fine-mesh sieve into the glass. Tuck a wedge of orange and lemon into the glass if you like. Store any unused tea in a covered container in the fridge.

¼ cup goji berries

4 tablespoons dried hibiscus flower

3 tablespoons agave nectar

2 cinnamon sticks

1 orange, cut into 8 wedges (optional)

1 lemon, cut into 8 wedges (optional)

PER SERVING: 29 calories, 0 g protein, 8 g carbohydrates, 0 g total fat (0 g saturated), 0 mg cholesterol, 0 g fiber, 0 mg sodium

Frozen Grape-Aid

Summers in Montauk are hot. The sun can be really intense all day and stays that way through the early evening. You have to stay hydrated at all costs, especially if you're diabetic, but at some point chugging all those endless bottles of water becomes downright tiresome. So my kitchen staff and I came up with a virgin sort of mojito-esque Kool-Aid thing. From their reactions—"Aww, sick! Oh man, that's rad! Sweet, dude!"—I think it was just the thing to beat the heat.

In a large resealable plastic bag, combine the grapes and blueberries and freeze overnight.

Have 4 glasses set and ready. In a beverage shaker, combine the mint leaves, frozen blueberries and grapes, and 4 of the lemon wedges. Grind together with a muddler or pestle until combined.

Divide the fruit mixture evenly among the 4 glasses. Top with crushed ice and club soda, garnish with a lemon wedge, and chill out.

1 cup halved red or green seedless grapes

½ cup blueberries

12 mint leaves

1 lemon, cut into 8 wedges

Crushed ice

1 liter club soda

PER SERVING: 41 calories, 1 g protein, 11 g carbohydrates, 0 g total fat (0 g saturated), 0 mg cholesterol, 1 g fiber, 1 mg sodium

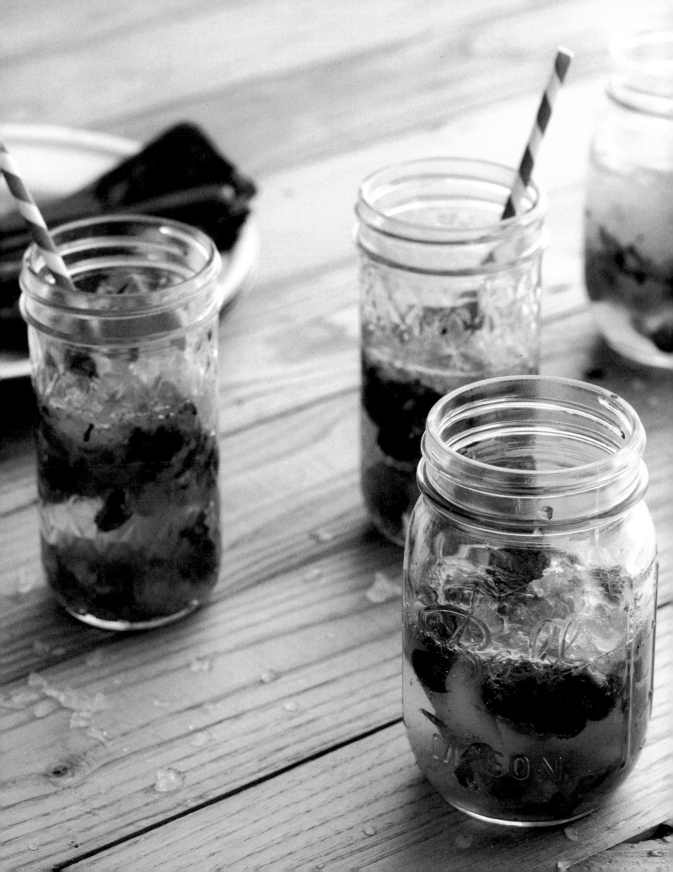

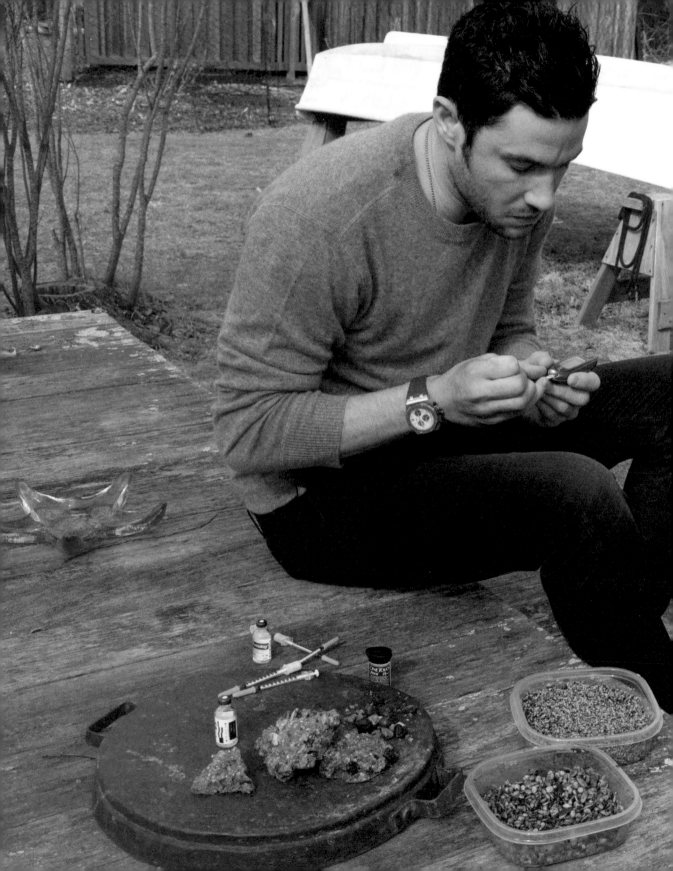

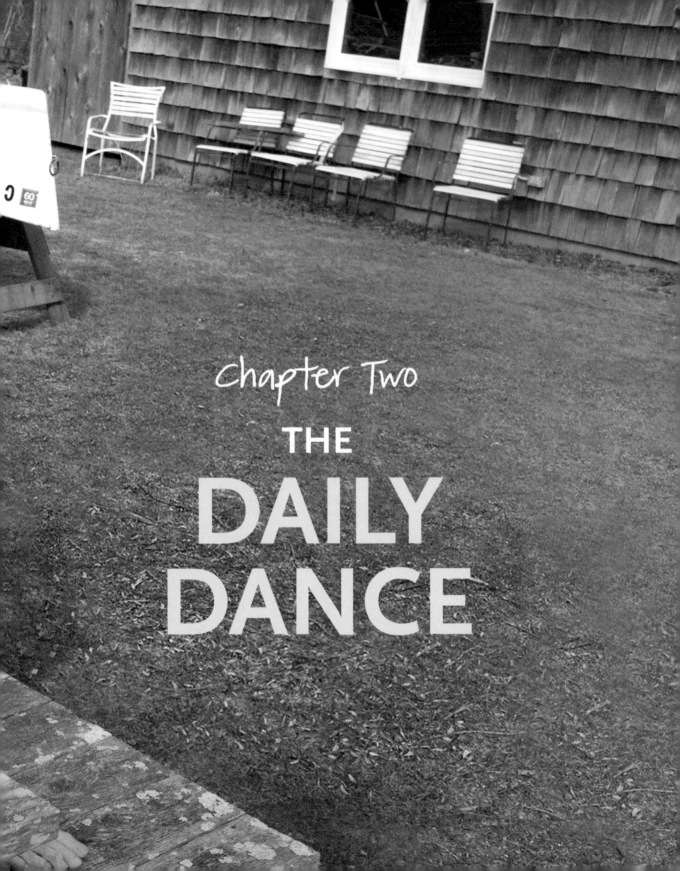

Chapter Two

THE
DAILY
DANCE

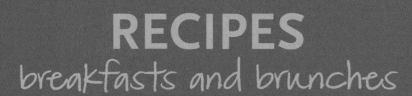

RECIPES
breakfasts and brunches

D ancers warm up at the barre or take a class every day to stay in shape. Diabetics have an equivalent discipline for staying healthy and safe. It consists of fueling up, cleaning up, and packing up before we set forth from Fortress Home. It's the daily dance, and getting this routine down will go a long way toward keeping you healthy—all day long.

GETTING GOING

It starts with the very first meal of the day. We've all been told a million times that breakfast is the most important meal of the day, but too often it's just a utilitarian meal aimed at getting the body in gear. No more. The granola, oatmeal, and pancakes in this chapter aren't the granola, oatmeal, or pancakes you grew up with by a long shot. And trust me when I say they are breakfasts that will supply power for a day of whatever you've got going, and they will send you off with your taste buds satisfied as well.

You may notice that some of these recipes are relatively high in carbs. I find that breakfast is the best time of day to take in the bulk of my daily carbs. It gives me a good boost of energy to get me going and coast on throughout the rest of the day.

Sometimes, though, you won't have time to put together a real breakfast, and in those instances, don't resort to a bagel from the coffee cart. Grab a yogurt and a fresh fruit—banana, apple, plum, whatever's in season—supplemented by a shot of açai extract and some vitamins.

I use açai a lot in the recipes in this book, and here's why. This small berry from the Amazon basin in Brazil packs an enormous amount of antioxidant power. With its fruity character and vaguely chocolate aftertaste, it works in both sweet and savory applications. Açai is also a renewable resource that can provide a sustainable livelihood for jungle dwellers without damaging the rain forest. So it's a food we can applaud for a lot of reasons and use to healthful *and* culinary effect.

As for vitamin supplements, I know that lots of people prefer to get all their nutrition from the food they eat. And in a perfect world, that's probably the best way to go. But given the nature of our disease, not to mention the busy lifestyles we all lead, we diabetics can use

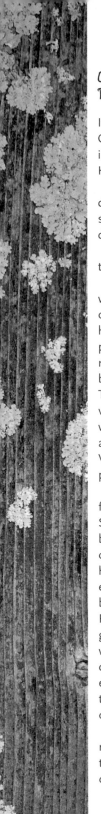

Oral Health: Dr. Gerry Says . . .

I've asked my good friend and dentist Dr. Gerry Curatola to explain why oral health is so important, whether you're diabetic or not. Here's what he has to say:

"Did you know that if you have dental disease—specifically, gum disease—you are seven times more likely to develop type 2 diabetes?

"By the same token, diabetics like Sam have to be extra careful about *getting* dental disease.

"Think of your mouth as a garden. In it grows what we call the oral biofilm, an aggregation of cells, which includes millions of bacteria that have an essential role in your ability to live—protecting you, aiding in digestion, and even manufacturing vitamins in the body. The oral biofilm is a perfectly balanced, healthy ecology. Throw that ecology off balance, and you become vulnerable to the formation of unhealthy plaque, which promotes tooth decay and gum disease and all that they can do to the rest of your body. What can throw the balance off? Four things in particular.

"Food is one—especially acid-promoting foods like refined carbs, sugars, and starches. Stress is another; it dries your mouth and can build up toxins. Not being fit can impede your circulation, which in turn can throw your mouth health off balance. It's why runners have an especially low incidence of gum disease: Their better circulation translates into better gums. Finally, chemicals—like those found in detergent-style toothpastes, alcohol-based mouthwashes, and home bleaching systems—can disturb, denature, and dehydrate the natural ecology of your mouth. It's like brushing your teeth with pesticides. So a key cornerstone of oral health is to 'go organic.'

"I hope you'll remember, as Sam does, that mouth disease is a silent, progressive killer, and that you can take charge of your health by taking charge of your mouth. Smile!"

an extra boost, and supplements are one good way to get it. Of course, as all the disclaimers say, you should check with your doctor about anything you ingest. I did, and I've been given the okay to take a daily multivitamin plus vitamins C and B.

CLEANING UP

Of course there's more to getting your day in gear than just heading out the door with a full stomach. You need to keep it clean, too, and by that I mean your teeth. For diabetics, oral health isn't just about having a pretty smile and white teeth. Actually, that's true for nondiabetics as well, but for diabetics, a clean mouth is really important. Research has shown what my dentist calls a "two-way street" between what happens in the mouth and its effect on the rest of the body—and vice versa. Our gums, teeth, and palate are so delicate and play such a vital role in our overall wellness that gum disease or any kind of oral-health issue can have very serious consequences on the heart, the digestion, the immune system, and all the other systems of the body. And, unfortunately, diabetics are more susceptible than most people to infections of the gums and mouth.

The difficulty we have regulating our blood sugar level can slow our circulation and lower our resistance to disease.

So for us, treating the mouth with the utmost respect is a matter of preventive health, and to me that means a mouth shower twice a day, every day. My practice is to clean with fluoride and floss my teeth in the morning and at night—and in between if and when I can. I know: Flossing blows. No one likes doing it. It's time-consuming and, let's face it, kind of gross. But if you're interested in your own overall wellness, it's one of the most important things you can do, and it offers a pretty rich payback in terms of health. Also, this twice-a-day mouth shower does give you a good-looking smile, and that never hurts.

PACKING UP

Okay. You're stoked, clean, and smiling—ready to grab your stuff and head out the door. "Grabbing your stuff" is another area where the discipline of a routine can keep you healthy and allow you to keep going through the day. Develop a system to make sure that you have all of the essentials on you at all times. There's no "give" on this. No exceptions. There is no time when you *may not need* to have your meter, test strips, insulin, syringe/pen, etc., on your person and within reach instantly. You *always* need your stuff. It really is a matter of life and death.

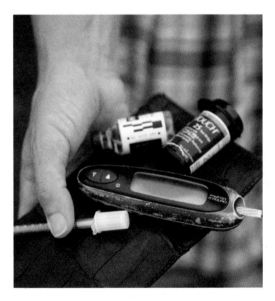

There's a pretty simple organizing principle for managing this: Put the diabetes supplies—your personal medical essentials—together, separated out from everything else, and always in the same place. The idea is not just that they're there, but that you *know* exactly where "there" is, and you know that you can just reach in and grab them as and when needed. With that kind of confidence, you can dance all day.

I was 14 when I figured out the pocket system that has served me well ever since, and I'm happy to share it here—although women may want to adapt it to the reality of skirts

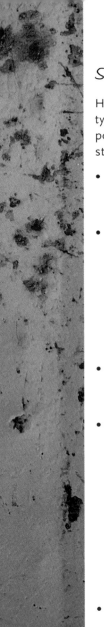

Supply and Demand

Here's my system—the supplies I typically keep on hand and the trigger points at which I know I need to re-stock them:

- **1,200 test strips last** me a month; 300 is the trigger number that tells me to restock.

- **150 syringes cover me** for a month—if I'm not on my pump, then I inject about five times a day, which adds up to about 150 injections a month; the truth is I'm always overstocked, so there's no trigger here at all—I just keep replenishing.

- **Two gallons of juice.** When one gallon is gone, that's the trigger to get another.

- **Three vials of insulin:** Lantus is my long-lasting insulin that I take at night—just one dose of 18 units. I also keep a few plastic bags of it prepacked in the fridge, ready for me to haul out at a moment's notice if I get a sudden invitation to hit the road, and I recommend you do the same. I reorder insulin when I start on the last vial—without fail.

- **A substantial stockpile of** either Pedialyte or another electrolyte-enhanced water; I keep these items in the pantry and get more when I see the supply dwindling. Don't be tempted to overstock Pedialyte, though, as it does carry an expiration date, which you should check periodically.

and purses. It's a simple, binary system: left pocket for medical, right for the personal stuff I feel naked without. The left-pocket contents are unchanged—in my case, three syringes, two bottles of insulin (and a third backup if the pants allow it), meter, and test strips. The right-pocket essentials change with the season, or the pants, or my mood; at the moment, they include lip balm, chewing gum, Lifesavers, and my wallet. But the left-pocket medical contents do not change.

Women carrying a handbag or tote—and some seem to be the size of miniature steamer trunks these days—could stash the left-pocket stuff in a zippered compartment dedicated to that purpose. Or keep it in a zippered cosmetics bag that you can put your hands on quickly and easily. One woman I know keeps her stuff in a furry bag so she can feel it among all the other stuff in her giganto tote. The principle, in any event, persists: medical essentials together, separate, always in the same place, easily accessible.

Backpacks are another good option. Those zippered compartments are secure repositories for additional backup syringes—at least, that's what I stuff in there—and the outside slots are the perfect place to stash a bottle of juice. I tend to fill my backpack with way too much stuff—laptop, iPod, workout clothes, a zillion chargers for all my electronics, notebooks, file folder, the book I think I'll read on the subway if I get a seat, etc.—but I always know my syringes are there if needed and there's a Naked Juice handy in case of low blood sugar. All I have to do is reach around and grab what I need.

The other must-have item to carry—in purse, pocket, briefcase, tote bag, or backpack—is a healthy snack. Choose one of the snacks offered on pages 23 to 32, or check out the list on page 157 for easy grab-and-go options. Portable and packable, these snacks can offer jolts of fortifying, satisfying energy all day long and a smarter alternative to anything you can pick up at the convenience store or corner coffee shop.

In this chapter, you'll find breakfasts that can fuel you and keep you going, as well as more substantial fare that would work for brunch. Make them as much a part your morning routine as checking your testing supplies and brushing your teeth, and you'll have made a good start on staying strong and healthy all day long.

YA GOTTA HAVE A SYSTEM

Having diabetes requires you to get organized—to build a system and stick to it. It's essential for managing the disease. And home is the headquarters for your system; it's the source of the supplies that keep you healthy and the place where you manage the disease every day.

The system should consist of the supplies you keep on hand and some sort of tickler mechanism that makes you go out and get more supplies before you run out—preferably well before you run out. Supplies to keep on hand include insulin, syringes, strips, and

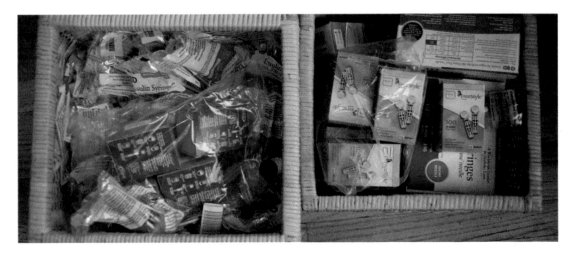

meters, of course, but also the items you know you may need to reach for if you begin to feel unwell or "off."

It's a good idea to designate a particular area for supplies. It could be a shelf in a closet or a basket on your bathroom countertop or a drawer in your bedroom. Whatever. Just a special space in your home where you know you can always find supplies. When you really need an injection, the last thing you want is to run around looking for a syringe and wondering where the hell you stashed that last batch you bought.

I keep my insulin supply in the top shelf of my fridge door. Then I've got one drawer in my bedroom for syringes and another for test strips, keystone strips, alcohol strips, and test meters. Nearby are shelves stocked with the supplies I keep on hand for when I fall into a low: sugar-free cough syrups, aspirin, Pedialyte, diet ginger ale, and Vitaminwater. These items are key for me, and I need to be able to reach out for one or all of them whenever I may be feeling sluggish, stressed, overworked, overtired, hungover, or sick with flu. As every diabetic knows, our disease makes it very hard to control an upset stomach or nausea; put bluntly, you sometimes can't stop puking—until and unless you find the right elixir. For me, it has always been diet ginger ale with bitters; it's what my mother gave me as a kid, and I still use it today when I'm feeling the funk. So, as you can imagine, having a good supply on hand is essential.

Part two of the system is the tickler mechanism—something besides just your good intentions to ensure that these drawers and shelves are always fully stocked and ready to go. There's a really good reason for this: Nothing is worse than having an upset stomach or a bout of nausea and crawling in agony over to the designated place where you keep the diet ginger ale only to find that somebody drank the last can, so you can't calm your stomach. Pedialyte is great for preventing dehydration if you've been vomiting. When I need Pedialyte, I really need it; I sip it slowly over the course of the day while eating bananas for sustenance. So if it's not there on the shelves when I need it, that's bad.

Lesson: Tedious as it may seem, you need a mechanism that forces you to restock your supplies—a number for each supply item that you've decided is the launching point for resupply. Only three ginger ales left? Buy more. Down to 200 strips? Now's the time to reorder. It's easier to be prepared, to keep checking supplies and restocking them, as needed—annoying as that may seem—than to get caught short.

I tend to rely on the Internet for ordering most supplies because it's far more economical—maybe one-tenth of what you pay over the counter. Of course, in this, as in just about everything in life, timing counts. If you're ordering insulin online, you've got to sync the prescription timing and the ordering and delivery timing. Ditto for strips and syringes—for everything. Getting it right, while not rocket science, can be a bit time-consuming. Which is precisely why I tend to put it off sometimes.

And then one day you find yourself caught without the supplies you need and forking over as much as $1.75 per strip at the local pharmacy—versus about three cents per strip online.

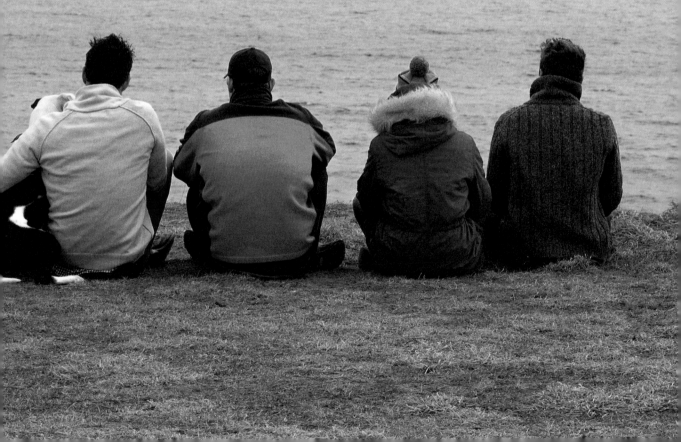

After you've paid the premium for being forgetful or lazy or too busy a couple of times, you'll see that it truly does make sense to keep on top of your supplies, and be proactive about looking ahead to your future needs. There's no alternative.

Of course emergencies like that happen to all of us. They shake you out of your lethargy so you get on your toes and check that supply shelf regularly and carefully. But the day is going to come again when you forget to look at the shelf or you put it off, and so it goes. Pay and move on—preferably without beating yourself up about it too much.

Again, it's all just part of the daily dance, putting a framework in place that keeps me prepared for the unexpected and sets me up to start the day on the best possible note. Any of the great breakfast recipes on the pages that follow will do the same for you.

TEAMMATES

It's essential to find a pharmacy—and a pharmacist—you can rely on. Nobody plays this game alone, and a home team backing you up in the dugout is essential. My guy in New York is the nicest man on the planet. Among other things, I know he is going to be in my corner when it's three o'clock on a Saturday afternoon and I am in a rush to get somewhere to start cooking and I run into the store, spilling my latte all over the place and telling him I'm in a bind and need a prescription filled. If Scotty is not in my corner at a moment like that, then I am, in the immortal words of Mr. Jagger, "between a rock and a hard place"—not a good place to be. I'm at his mercy. So the fact that Scotty has never let me down is amazingly valuable to me, and I make a point of letting him know that any and every way I can.

For me, it's simple: A diabetic needs a good pharmacist the same way a chef needs a good fishmonger. I treat Scotty like my fishmonger—with the greatest respect. In both cases, it goes a long way.

Almond Milk: Good for You

Almond milk contains more nutrients than any other dairy milk alternative. In fact, its health benefits match those of dairy choices. It's a particularly good alternative for those with soy and lactose sensitivities. Almond milk offers a lucky seven health benefits:

1. WEIGHT MANAGEMENT

Plain almond milk without added sugars or flavoring contains 40 calories per 8-ounce serving. So if you're looking to lose weight or maintain a low weight, that's a nice, light touch on whatever daily calorie total you're shooting for. Keep in mind as you prepare your morning cereal that a number of the other milk alternatives contain more sugars than the cereal you're pouring it on.

2. HEART HEALTH

Almond milk contains no cholesterol and only 5 milligrams of sodium per serving. Obviously, that's good for heart health. In addition, a serving of almond milk contains 150 milligrams of potassium, which is particularly beneficial in promoting healthy blood pressure—another plus for the health of your heart.

3. BLOOD SUGAR–FRIENDLY

Unlike other milk alternatives, almond milk contains only 8 grams of carbohydrate per serving, and the 7 grams of sugars that make up this carbohydrate content have a limited effect on our blood sugar levels. Why? Unlike simple sugars, which lack nutrients and which our bodies tend to store as fat, these sugars are low on the glycemic index, so our bodies fully digest them and use them as energy. This makes almond milk a boon for diabetics—and mighty friendly to nondiabetics as well.

4. BONE HEALTH

With 30 percent of the daily value for calcium and 25 percent of the RDA for vitamin D, almond milk contributes to bone strength at any age. Moreover, it contains magnesium, which helps the body absorb calcium. The vitamin D content also helps improve immunity and cell function; it may even decrease the risk of osteoporosis and in some studies has been shown to slow Alzheimer's disease.

5. SKIN CARE

Every serving of pure almond milk contains 50 percent of the recommended daily intake of vitamin E, an antioxidant that is the primary regulatory nutrient for skin health.

6. EYE HEALTH

The vitamin A found in almond milk helps keep our eyes functioning properly—especially when it comes to adjusting to differences in light.

7. MORE MUSCLE POWER

Even though almond milk contains only 1 gram of protein per serving, it does contain B vitamins and other muscle-regulating nutrients such as iron. These nutrients help muscles absorb and use protein for energy, growth, and repair.

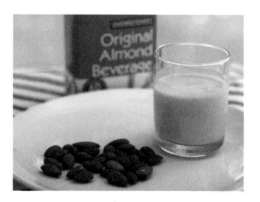

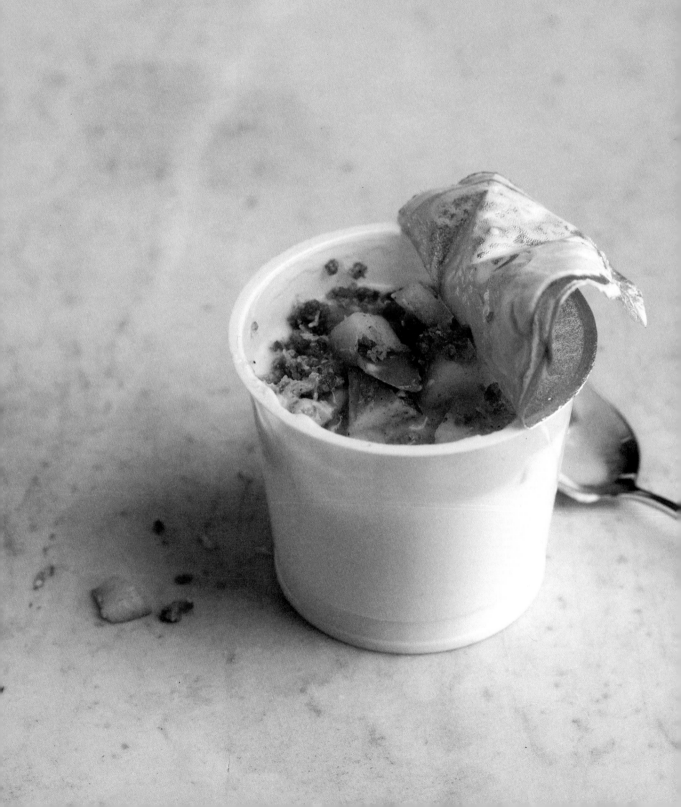

Yogurt with Pear and Coconut

Parfait is what kids order in restaurants, right? And their eyes get huge when the waiter puts that tall glass with the short stem in front of them, and there's all that lavish sweetness spiraling up and up in swirls of colors in the glass. Want to feel that way again? Here you go—the best, and so low-fat and low-calorie you can enjoy it without guilt.

In a medium bowl, combine the lemon juice, coconut, graham cracker crumbs, cereal, sweetener, and cinnamon.

Peel, core, and finely chop the pears. Spoon the yogurt into 4 bowls and top with the fruit and coconut mixture or sprinkle directly onto each individual container of yogurt.

Note: This recipe can do double-duty as a dessert if you serve it up parfait-style. Spoon ⅛ of the pears into the bottom of each of 4 bowls or parfait glasses. Add ⅛ of the cereal mixture, then ½ cup of yogurt. Repeat with the remaining pears, cereal mixture, and yogurt.

PER SERVING: 265 calories, 15 g protein, 38 g carbohydrates, 8 g total fat (6 g saturated), 8 mg cholesterol, 6 g fiber, 157 mg sodium

Juice of 1 lemon

⅓ cup unsweetened shredded coconut

2 tablespoons graham cracker crumbs

½ cup Grape-Nuts or granola cereal

1 tablespoon granulated stevia extract, or to taste

1 teaspoon ground cinnamon

2 ripe Bosc pears, slightly firm to the touch

3 cups 2% plain Greek yogurt

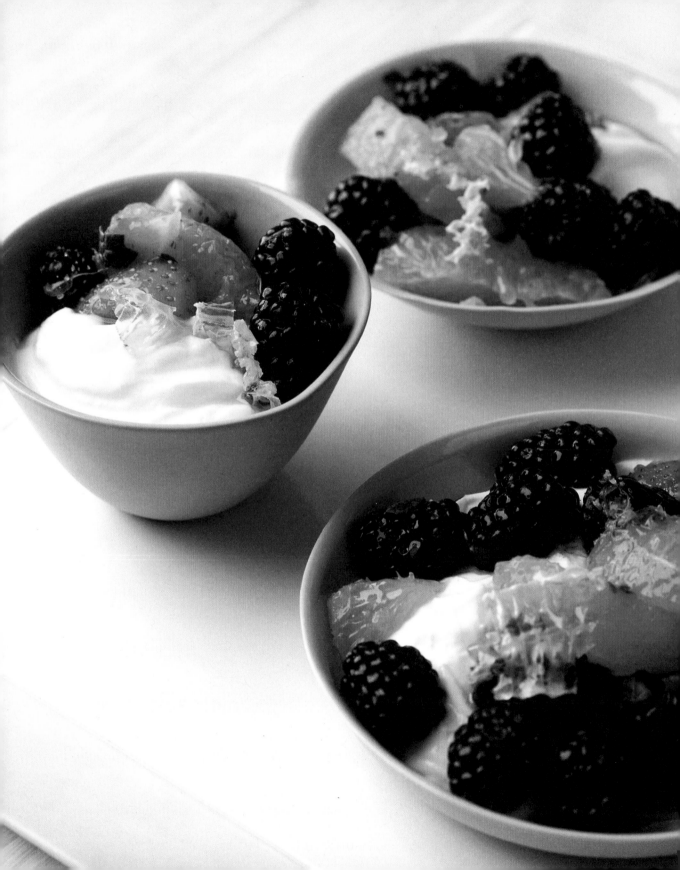

Blackberry Salad with mint and Honeycomb

4

I love to start the day with fresh fruit; it's perfect for whatever the day is going to bring: big meeting, relaxing morning, waves, or the gym—it doesn't matter. That first bite of a fresh-picked blackberry is the best of summer. The juice squirts down your lip and tastes just like heaven. Fresh blackberries with citrus, mint, and honeycomb come together to kill it in this anytime, anywhere fruit salad. And it's super easy to make. (If not blackberries, sub whatever seasonal berry or fruit that you can score locally. If the berry is in season and it's bought where it's grown, you can't go wrong, as we all know by now.)

Using a sharp knife, slice off the skin and pith from one of the grapefruits. Holding it over a medium bowl, cut between the membranes to release the grapefruit segments, and add them to the bowl. Squeeze the membranes to get all the juice. Grate 1 teaspoon of zest from the second grapefruit and juice the grapefruit into the bowl. Add the blackberries and strawberries and toss gently with a rubber spatula to combine. Add the mint and gently toss again until it is well distributed.

Spoon ½ cup of yogurt into each of 4 bowls and top each serving with a spoonful or two of fruit and a bit of honeycomb.

2 **Ruby Red grapefruits**

2 **pints blackberries**

1 **cup quartered strawberries**

½ **cup loosely packed chopped fresh mint leaves**

2 **cups 2% plain organic Greek yogurt**

4 **teaspoon-size scoops honeycomb**

PER SERVING: 199 calories, 12 g protein, 38 g carbohydrates, 3 g total fat (2 g saturated), 5 mg cholesterol, 11 g fiber, 40 mg sodium

Egg whites for One with Blueberry and Cinnamon

 It's hard to believe one breakfast can contain so many good-for-you ingredients. Studies show that as little as half a teaspoon of cinnamon per day improves insulin sensitivity and blood glucose control. That, in turn, can help control weight and decrease the risk of heart disease. The same studies have also noted cinnamon's role in improving triglyceride levels, blood pressure, and LDL cholesterol. And everyone knows what a nutritional superstar the blueberry is.

The whites are cholesterol-free (it's the yolks that contain almost an entire day's worth of cholesterol). Plus, 1 cup of egg whites has 26 grams of protein. And egg whites are so versatile to cook with. I eat them constantly—at least four times a week.

I know, though: Apart from the health benefits, these three ingredients sounds weird as hell together. But trust me, they combine so well it's crazy.

In a medium bowl, whisk together the egg whites, milk, cinnamon, salt, and pepper until smooth and frothy.

In a small nonstick skillet, heat the oil over medium-high heat. Add the egg white mixture and as it begins to set, use a spatula to lift the edges and let the undercooked egg run from the middle to the bottom of the pan. When the egg whites are set, remove from the heat and slide them onto a plate. Top with the blueberries and sprinkle with the lemon zest.

PER SERVING: 166 calories, 11 g protein, 10 g carbohydrates, 10 g total fat (1 g saturated), 0 mg cholesterol, 3 g fiber, 508 mg sodium

3 **egg whites**

2 **tablespoons almond milk**

1 **teaspoon ground cinnamon**

¼ **teaspoon fine sea salt**

½ **teaspoon freshly ground black pepper**

2 **teaspoons olive oil**

¼ **cup blueberries**

1 **teaspoon grated lemon zest**

Soft-Cooked Eggs with Yellow Squash and Broccoli Rabe Pesto

 6

This is one of those do-right, wins-every-time, trustworthy egg dishes. Picky, affected hipster types, preteens, moms: Everybody likes this. Sometimes, after a night of drinking with friends, we all end up at someone's house with everyone begging me to cook. Since eggs are pretty much a staple in everyone's fridge, it often ends up being some variation of this dish. This version is an homage to my friend Natalie; she's a veg head, so when I cook at her place, the random squash and the occasional whatnot ends up in there. Feel free to use what you find in your crisper drawer.

To make the pesto: Bring a small pot of generously salted water to a boil over medium-high heat. Add the broccoli rabe and cook until fork-tender, about 1 minute. Drain into a colander and rinse under cold water for 45 seconds to stop the cooking and retain the bright green color. Set aside to cool slightly.

In a blender or food processor, combine the roasted garlic, almonds, agave nectar, lemon juice, cooled broccoli rabe, and ¼ cup water. Puree the mixture until smooth. With the machine running, gradually stream in the extra-virgin olive oil and blend until combined. If the consistency is too thick, add water accordingly, keeping the blender on low. Once the pesto is to your liking, transfer it to a small bowl and fold in the Parmesan with a rubber spatula. You will need only 3 tablespoons of pesto for this recipe, so you can freeze the extra or keep it in the fridge in an airtight container for up to 1 week.

To cook the eggs: In a large bowl, combine the eggs, milk, squash, and 3 tablespoons of the pesto.

In a large nonstick skillet, heat the olive oil over medium-high heat. Add the egg mixture and reduce the heat to low. As the eggs begin to set, add the basil and scallions and use a spatula to lift the edges and let the undercooked egg run from the middle to the bottom of the pan. As soon as the eggs are set, remove the pan from the heat and serve the eggs hot.

PER SERVING: 414 calories, 18 g protein, 17 g carbohydrates, 31 g total fat (5 g saturated), 303 mg cholesterol, 3 g fiber, 224 mg sodium

BROCCOLI RABE PESTO

Salt

- ½ bunch broccoli rabe (½ pound), tough stem ends trimmed
- 5 cloves Roasted Garlic (page 93), lightly mashed
- 1 cup sliced almonds, toasted in a dry skillet
- 2 tablespoons agave nectar

  Juice of 2 lemons
- ⅓ cup extra-virgin olive oil
- ¼ cup grated Parmesan cheese

EGGS

- 10 cage-free organic eggs
- ⅓ cup almond milk or soy milk
- 1 yellow squash, cut in ¼-inch-thick half-moons
- 1 tablespoon olive oil
- ¼ cup thinly sliced fresh basil leaves
- 4 scallions, thinly sliced

Peas with Mint and Soft Poached Eggs

I meet my friend Joel once a month for breakfast at the Noho Star and I always get the same thing: scrambled eggs with peas and tomatoes. Here, I have swapped poached eggs for scrambled, and I amped up the flavor by adding some fresh mint. Feel free to swap out the green peas for snap peas or pea sprouts if you like. When the yolk breaks, the dish goes from great to stellar in seconds.

Bring a large pot of water to a boil over medium-high heat. Blanch the peas in the boiling water until they turn bright green, about 25 seconds. Drain in a colander and run them under cold water for 30 seconds to stop the cooking. Set aside.

In a large saucepan, combine 4 cups of water with the vinegar, salt, and 1 tablespoon of the lemon juice. Bring the mixture to a rapid simmer over medium-high heat. Crack the eggs on the side of the pan and gently slip them into the water. Let the eggs settle into the liquid and cook until coagulated, about 3 minutes. Using a slotted spoon, transfer the cooked eggs to a shallow plate.

In a large skillet, heat the oil over medium-high heat. Add the celery, onion, and garlic and cook until translucent, 2 to 3 minutes. Add the mint, tomatoes, and blanched peas. Season to taste with salt and pepper and sprinkle with the lemon zest and juice. Toss well to combine.

Divide the pea mixture among 4 plates and top with 2 poached eggs per serving.

PER SERVING: 320 calories, 17 g protein, 19 g carbohydrates, 19 g total fat (4 g saturated), 360 mg cholesterol, 5 g fiber, 480 mg sodium

- 2 cups shelled fresh green peas
- ¼ cup distilled white vinegar
- 1 tablespoon fine sea salt
- 1 tablespoon lemon juice plus grated zest and juice of 1 lemon
- 8 organic cage-free eggs
- 3 tablespoons olive oil
- 1 celery rib, thinly sliced crosswise on the diagonal
- 1 small yellow onion, finely diced
- 2 garlic cloves, smashed and finely chopped
- ½ cup hand-torn fresh mint leaves
- 2 heirloom tomatoes or medium vine-ripened tomatoes, coarsely chopped
- Salt and freshly ground black pepper

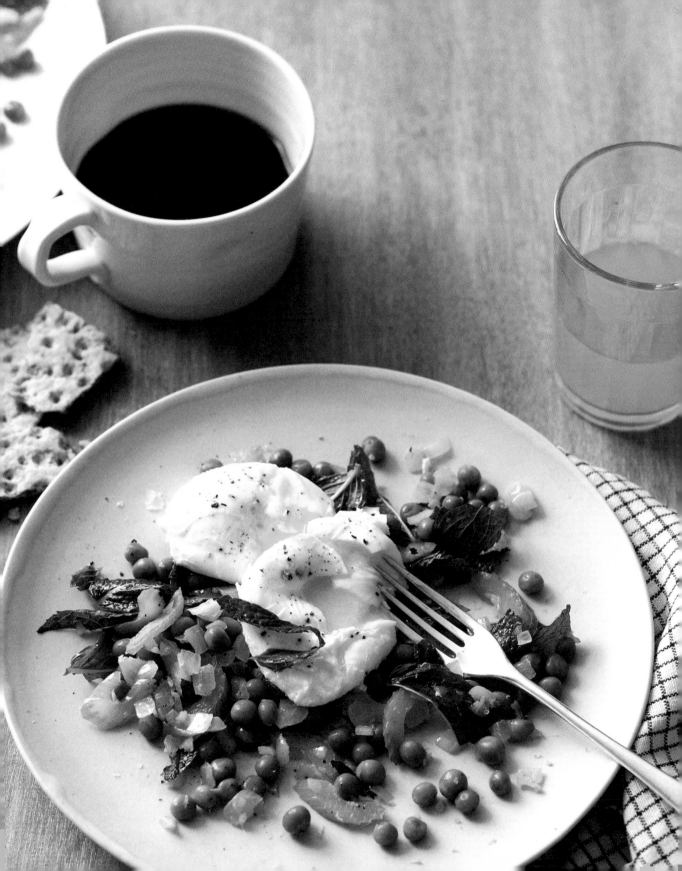

Baked Eggs with Chickpeas and Harissa

(4) Chickpeas are loaded with fiber. In fact, some studies show that eating chickpeas daily can begin to help regulate your blood sugar. By adding cinnamon to the chickpeas, you're really tapping into diabetes wellness. Now, making a baked egg correctly is an art form. Usually they're so overcooked they are as hard as a hockey puck. This is not good. No fear here. Make it my way a few times to master the technique, then change it up with any ingredients you like: Try black beans and tomatillos, couscous and stewed tomatoes—you get the idea.

Preheat the oven to 350°F. Grease four 6- to 8-ounce gratin dishes with cooking spray or butter.

In a medium bowl, combine the fresh tomato, canned tomatoes, chickpeas, arugula, thyme, almond milk, Parmesan, oil, harissa, and cinnamon. Mix together until well combined and season to taste with salt and pepper. Divide the mixture among the gratin dishes.

Crack 2 eggs over each gratin dish and bake until the eggs have set, 8 to 10 minutes. Remove from the oven and serve hot.

PER SERVING: 321 calories, 19 g protein, 18 g carbohydrates, 18 g total fat (5 g saturated), 366 mg cholesterol, 4 g fiber, 447 mg sodium

- 1 medium vine-ripened tomato, cut into 8 wedges
- ½ cup canned crushed San Marzano tomatoes
- 1 can (15 ounces) chickpeas, rinsed and drained
- ½ cup baby arugula
- Leaves from ¼ bunch fresh thyme
- ¼ cup almond milk
- 3 tablespoons grated Parmesan cheese
- 2 tablespoons olive oil
- 1 tablespoon harissa
- ½ teaspoon ground cinnamon
- Salt and freshly ground black pepper
- 8 cage-free organic eggs

Baked Eggs with Pancetta-Basil Marinara

 4

I first met baked eggs about 8 or 9 years ago at a li'l bistro in the Meatpacking District of downtown Manhattan. The bistro is now long gone, but I will never forget baked eggs with merguez sausage, harissa, and chickpeas, served piping hot in the skillet they were baked in. My version is a bit on the healthier side, but you can always add sausage or bacon if you like. Once you get hooked on these you will never go back to the boring scramble. Hot and bubbly with a perfectly runny yolk: heaven!

In a medium saucepan, heat the oil over medium-high heat. Add the garlic, onion, carrots, and pancetta and cook, stirring frequently, until the pancetta is lightly browned, 2 to 3 minutes. Drain off and discard half of the juice from the can of tomatoes, then add the tomatoes and remaining juice to the pan. Bring the sauce to a boil. Reduce to a simmer and cook for at least 30 minutes or up to 2 hours to concentrate the flavors. Just before serving, stir in the thyme and basil and season lightly with salt and pepper.

Preheat the oven to 350°F. Grease four 8-ounce gratin dishes with nonstick cooking spray or butter. Place the dishes on a baking sheet.

Fill each gratin dish two-thirds full with marinara, then crack 1 egg into each gratin dish. Bake until the eggs have set, 8 to 10 minutes. Serve hot.

2 tablespoons olive oil

4 garlic cloves, smashed and chopped

¼ cup diced yellow onion

2 carrots, finely diced

1 ounce pancetta, diced

1 can (28 ounces) crushed San Marzano tomatoes

2 tablespoons fresh thyme leaves

½ cup hand-torn fresh basil leaves

Salt and freshly ground black pepper

4 cage-free organic eggs

PER SERVING: 258 calories, 13 g protein, 21 g carbohydrates, 14 g total fat (3 g saturated), 223 mg cholesterol, 3 g fiber, 1,001 mg sodium

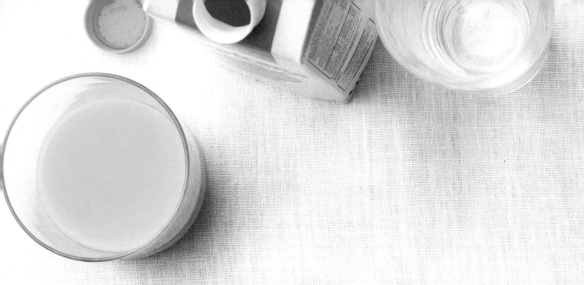

chickpea and Cherry Frittata

Don't be put off by the seeming incongruity of the ingredients in this egg dish. It makes a statement—it's big, sort of out of line, shapely to look at, and bold flavored. Bang this one down in the warm skillet and put out some forks and napkins and red wine and watch how a group of intensely hungover adults react. They'll go from "Oh my head hurts, oh I want my bed" to "Oh, wait: What's that in the pan? Hey, is that Pinot from Oregon?" before you know it.

Preheat the oven to 350°F.

In a medium bowl, mix together the eggs, chickpeas, cherries, goat cheese, almond milk, thyme, agave nectar, and cream of tartar.

In a medium ovenproof skillet, heat the oil over medium heat. Pour the egg mixture into the skillet and cook for 2 minutes without stirring. Transfer the skillet to the oven and bake until the eggs are puffed and set in the middle, 30 to 35 minutes. Let the frittata cool for 5 to 10 minutes.

With a rubber spatula, gently work the frittata out of the pan and transfer it to a cutting board. Cut the frittata into wedges and serve warm, garnished with the mint.

PER SERVING: 201 calories, 11 g protein, 14 g carbohydrates, 11 g total fat (4 g saturated), 191 mg cholesterol, 2 g fiber, 189 mg sodium

- 8 cage-free organic eggs
- 1 can (15 ounces) chickpeas, rinsed and drained
- 1 cup chopped fresh cherries or ½ cup chopped dried cherries
- 4 ounces goat cheese, crumbled
- ¼ cup almond milk
- 1 tablespoon chopped fresh thyme leaves
- 2 tablespoons agave nectar
- 1 teaspoon cream of tartar
- 1 tablespoon olive oil
- ¼ cup loosely packed hand-torn fresh mint leaves

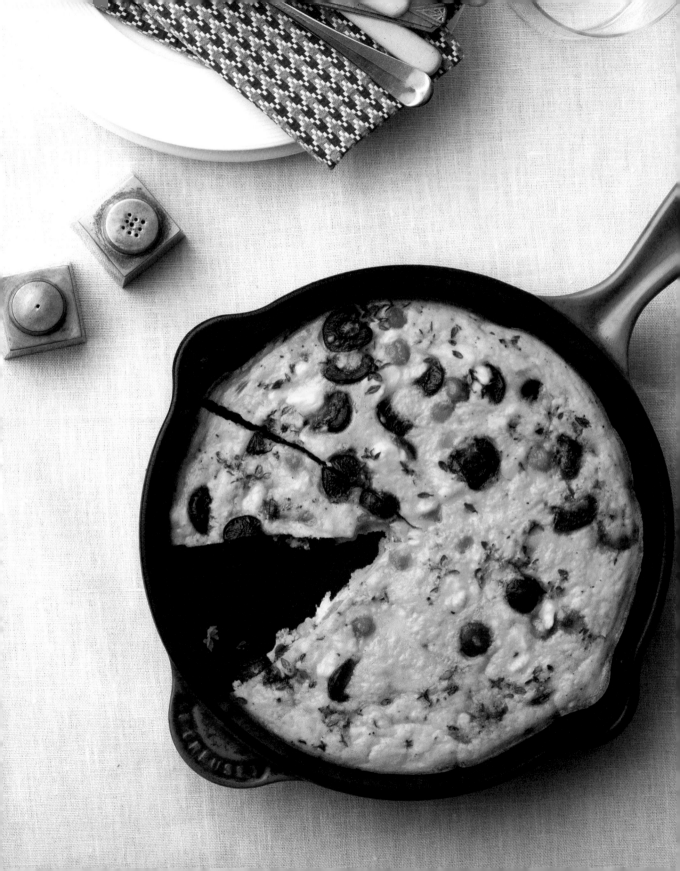

Pickled Peach and Walnut Pancakes

These pancakes can constitute the most satisfying brunch you've ever had, giving a whole new meaning to the Sweet Life. If your mouth puckers up at the thought of pickled peaches, think again.

To make the pickled peaches: In a large airtight container, combine the agave nectar, vinegar, 1 cup cold water, the lemon zest and juice, sweetener, and allspice. Add the peaches, cover, and refrigerate for at least 30 minutes or overnight.

To make the pancakes: In a large bowl, combine the flour, sweetener, baking powder, baking soda, and walnuts. Mix until just combined. In a small bowl, lightly beat the eggs. Whisk in the almond milk, buttermilk, applesauce, and agave nectar until combined. Slowly mix the milk mixture into the flour mixture until just barely combined—do not overmix.

Heat a medium skillet or griddle over medium-high heat and coat it with cooking spray. Working in batches, drop ⅓ cup of batter per pancake onto the skillet and cook until bubbles appear on the surface. Then flip the pancakes and cook through. Repeat with the rest of the batter, making 8 to 10 hot cakes.

Serve the pancakes topped with the pickled peaches.

PER SERVING: 503 calories, 19 g protein, 30 g carbohydrates, 38 g total fat (4 g saturated), 162 mg cholesterol, 8 g fiber, 391 mg sodium

PICKLED PEACHES

- 3 tablespoons agave nectar
- 2 tablespoons cider vinegar
- Grated zest and juice of 1 lemon
- 1 tablespoon granulated stevia extract, or to taste
- 1½ teaspoons ground allspice
- 3 peaches, peeled and pitted, each sliced into 12 wedges

PANCAKES

- 1¾ cups almond flour
- 1 tablespoon granulated stevia extract, or to taste
- 1 teaspoon baking powder
- ½ teaspoon baking soda
- ½ cup chopped walnuts
- 3 cage-free organic eggs
- ¾ cup almond milk
- ½ cup low-fat buttermilk
- ½ cup unsweetened applesauce

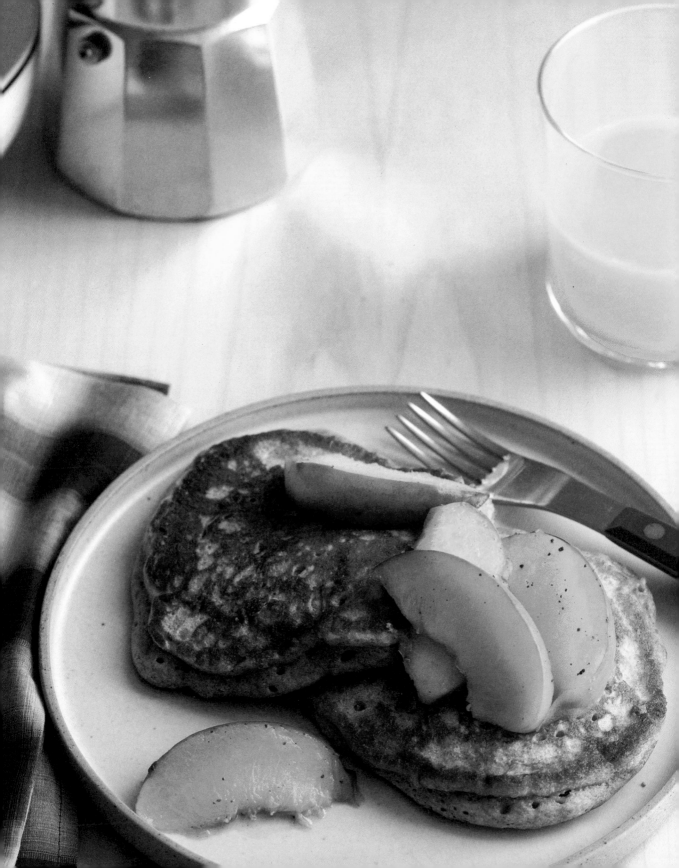

Lemon Ricotta Hot Cakes

 6–8

It seems like every time I turn around someone is saying, "Oh yeah, so-and-so's lemon ricotta cakes are the best thing EVER," and they can get kind of emotional about it, which I totally understand—they are awesome just about any way you make them. But to put an end to the debate and controversy, I offer these lemon ricotta hot cakes—truly *the* most perfect way to start the day. Imagine: It's Saturday morning, you're in bed, and in walks (insert name here) with a plate of these good cakes with a fried egg on top. Yikes—good eating.

In a large bowl, whisk together the lemon zest and juice, ricotta, milk, almond milk, agave nectar, applesauce, sour cream, and egg yolks. In a medium bowl, mix together the flour, sweetener, baking powder, and baking soda. Add the flour mixture to the ricotta mixture and mix until combined. The batter will be slightly lumpy.

In a small bowl, whisk the egg whites until they form soft peaks. Using a rubber spatula, fold the beaten egg whites into the batter.

Heat a medium skillet or griddle over medium-high heat and coat it with cooking spray. Working in batches, drop ⅓ cup of batter per hot cake onto the skillet and cook until bubbles appear on the surface. Then flip the hot cakes and cook through. Repeat with the rest of the batter, making 8 to 10 hot cakes.

PER SERVING: 155 calories, 7 g protein, 24 g carbohydrates, 4 g total fat (2 g saturated), 112 mg cholesterol, 3 g fiber, 360 mg sodium

Grated zest and juice of 2 lemons

1 **cup whole-milk ricotta cheese**

1 **cup whole milk**

3 **tablespoons almond milk**

1 **tablespoon agave nectar**

2 **tablespoons unsweetened applesauce**

1 **tablespoon reduced-fat sour cream**

3 **organic cage-free organic eggs, separated**

1 **cup whole wheat flour**

1 **tablespoon granulated stevia extract**

1 **teaspoon baking powder**

1 **teaspoon baking soda**

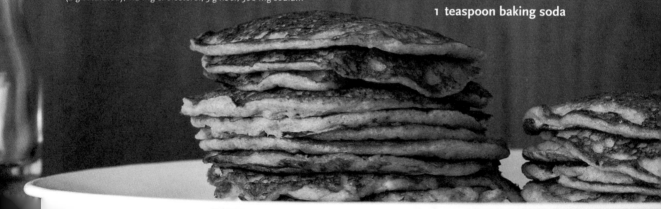

Vanilla Whole Grain French Toast

 6

Okay, French toast is clearly not the most diabetic-friendly breakfast around, but once in a blue moon, if you have a big day of outdoor activities planned, it's worth the splurge. This version is slightly sweet, so you won't miss the syrup.

In a medium bowl, whisk together the eggs, almond milk, agave nectar, vanilla, cinnamon, and allspice until well combined. Pour the mixture into a shallow bowl. Dip the bread slices in the egg mixture, turning to coat well.

Heat a medium skillet or griddle over medium-high heat and coat it with cooking spray. Cook each egg-soaked bread half until golden brown, 4 to 5 minutes per side. Serve warm, 3 half-slices per person.

PER SERVING: 165 calories, 7 g protein, 28 g carbohydrates, 4 g total fat (1 g saturated), 143 mg cholesterol, 8 g fiber, 186 mg sodium

4 **cage-free organic eggs, lightly beaten**

¾ cup **vanilla almond milk**

2 tablespoons **agave nectar**

1 teaspoon **pure vanilla extract**

1 teaspoon **ground cinnamon**

½ teaspoon **ground allspice**

9 **slices whole grain bread, halved**

Almond and Açai Steel-Cut Oatmeal

 Steel-cut oats are much lower on the glycemic index than most flavored instant oatmeals and are therefore a great way to keep blood sugar levels low. Yes, the steel-cut oats cost more and have a longer cooking time, but for me, the crunchy texture and heartier taste alone make this breakfast dish worth the price and the wait. Flavoring the oats with super foods like almonds and açai boosts this dish even further, arming you with necessary fiber, vitamins, and minerals for natural energy that will last all day.

Bring 3 cups of water to a boil in a pot.

Meanwhile, in a large saucepan, melt the butter over low heat. Add the oats and stir them constantly until toasted, 2 to 3 minutes.

Add the boiling water to the oats and bring to a simmer. Cook, stirring constantly, until thickened, 15 to 20 minutes.

Mix in the almond milk, agave nectar, açai powder, and toasted almonds. Serve hot.

1 teaspoon unsalted butter

1 cup steel-cut oats

1 cup plus 2 tablespoons almond milk

2 tablespoons agave nectar

2 tablespoons açai powder

¼ cup sliced almonds, toasted in the oven

PER SERVING: 254 calories, 8 g protein, 38 g carbohydrates, 10 g total fat (3 g saturated), 3 mg cholesterol, 5 g fiber, 51 mg sodium

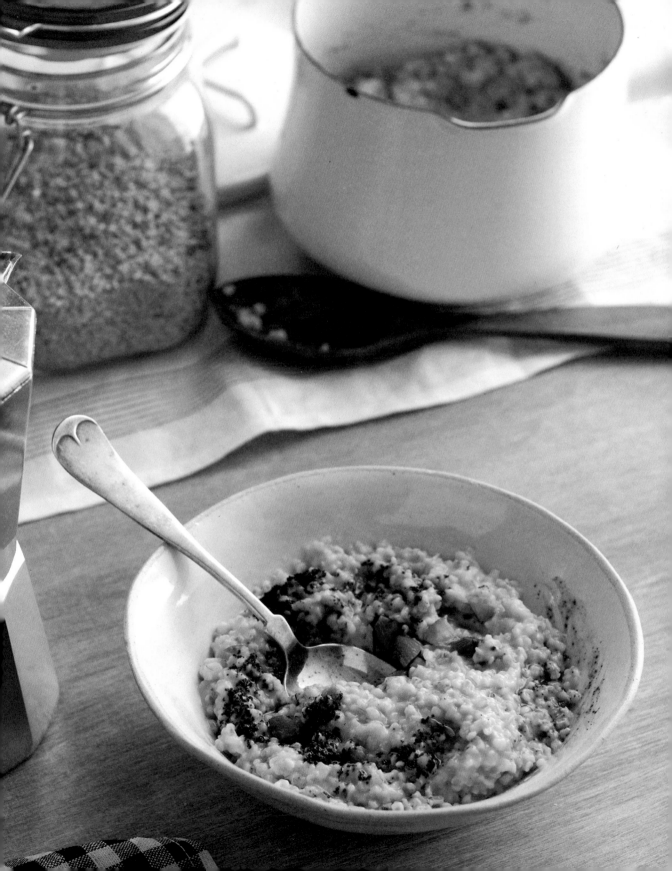

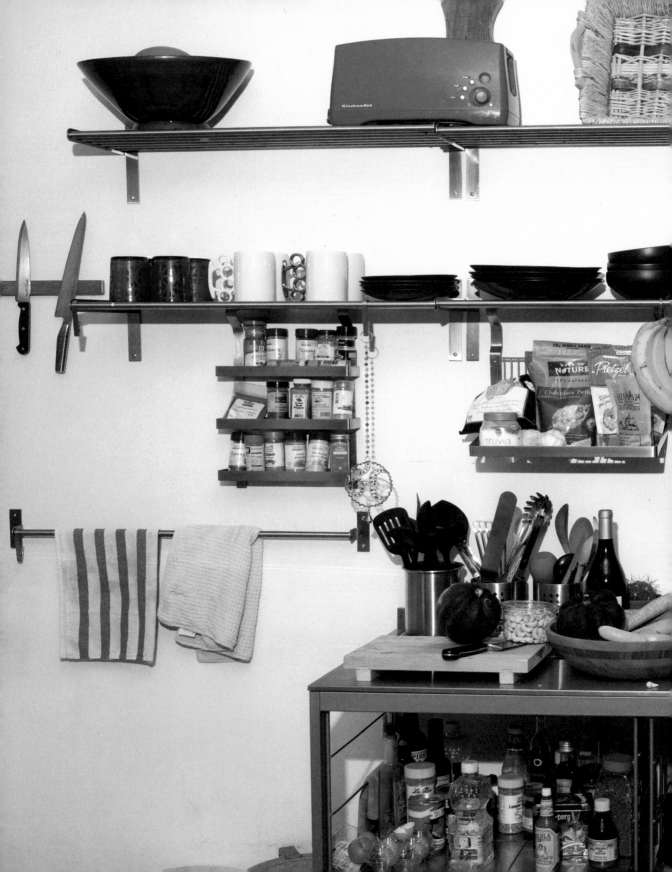

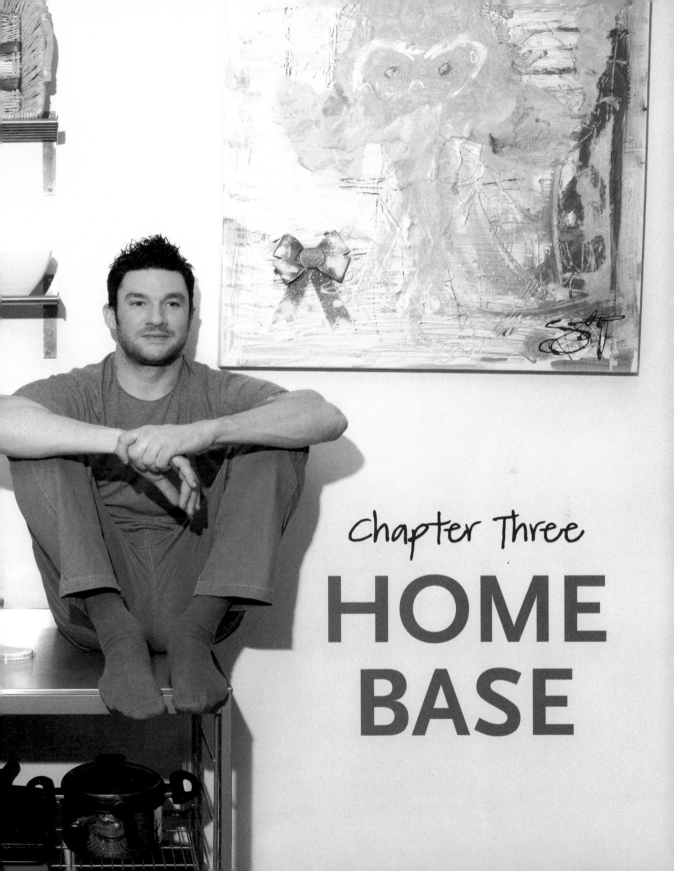

Chapter Three

HOME
BASE

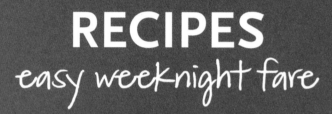

RECIPES
easy weeknight fare

T he Sweet Life begins at home.

After all, home is your haven, your refuge, the headquarters where your health gets recharged and—always—the place where you're most comfortable. That means that all the things we diabetics have to do as a matter of course—stay balanced, think ahead, pay attention to the way we eat—need to be second nature for us at home. And that's probably a good model for nondiabetics as well.

Creating a safe, healthy space at home is pretty simple: You want to eliminate what's not good for you, bring in what is good for you, and make it a place where you can quickly and easily put together a healthy, delicious meal. After all, it's a lot easier to eat well when you know everything that goes into a dish, and most of the time it tastes better, too.

WHAT TO KEEP OUT

What do I mean by keeping out what's not good for you? It's not just about what's in your fridge. Take, for example, smoking. I'm friends with many smokers. I wish they wouldn't smoke because I care about them, but that's their business; I just don't allow it in my home.

Stress is another example. I'm big on keeping the stress levels in my home on an even keel—a *low* even keel. Stress is a real danger for diabetics. For one thing, stress can send your blood sugar level flying all over the place—mostly way up, but too far down as well. For another thing, stress can throw off your life in general—to the point where you may forget or not care about checking your blood or planning a good meal or going to the gym today, or this week, or ever. So stress is definitely something to be managed, and the last place you want to be stressed out is at home.

That means if you live on a truck route where the tractor trailers run all day, or if your neighbors turn up the volume on *Simpsons* reruns late at night, or there's a tree on your lawn with a long branch hanging right over your roof, you need to take action or move. Call your congressman about the truck route, take your neighbors to court, pay an expert to cut the branch—or even the whole tree—or find a new address. Your home should be a place where you feel safe and comfortable—not stressed out.

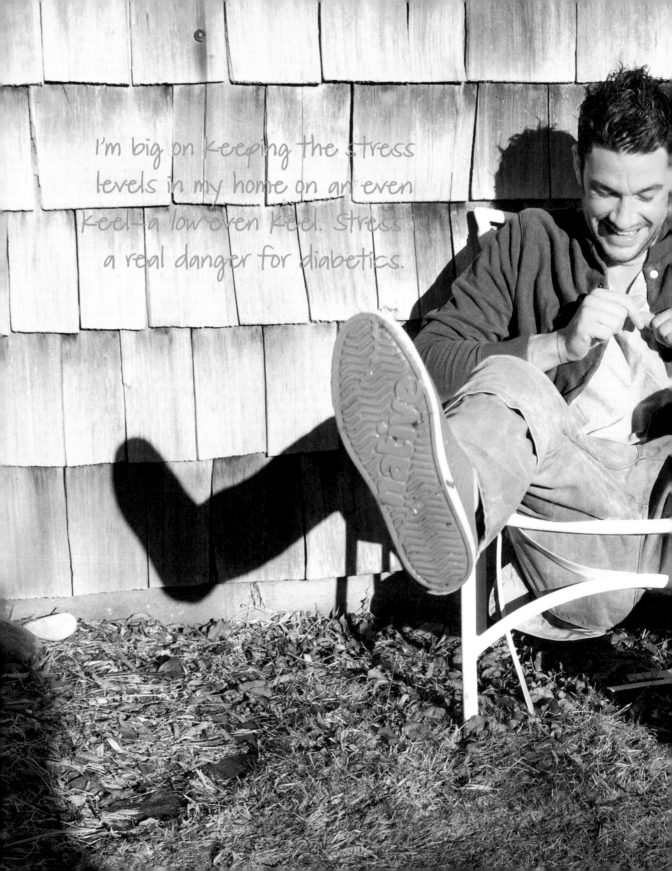

I'm big on keeping the stress levels in my home on an even keel—a low even keel. Stress a real danger for diabetics.

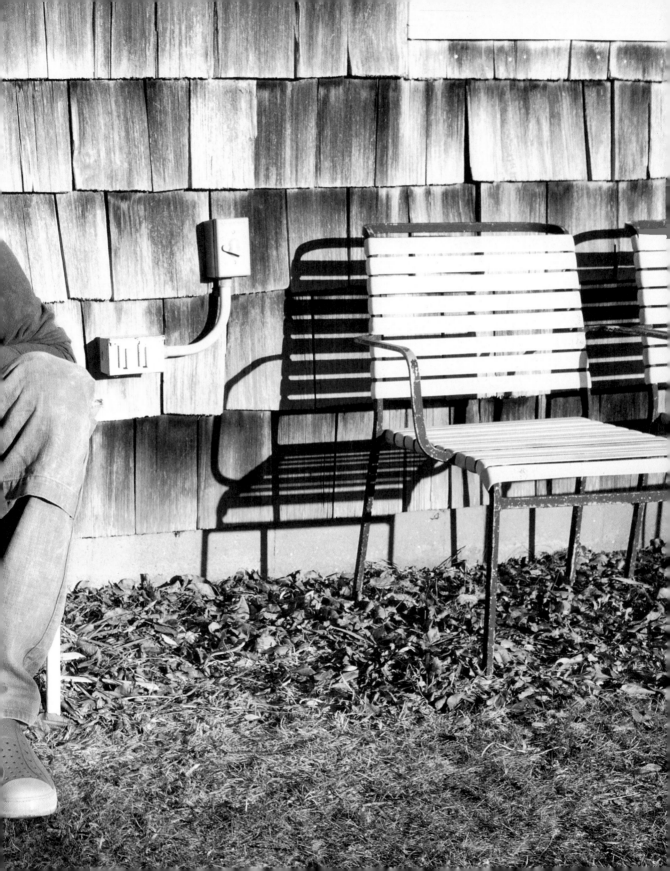

Sometimes, you can only keep stress down by keeping it out. I get pretty adamant about that where guests are concerned. If you're visiting me, you need to be in a nonstress-inducing mode—even an antistress-inducing mode—or you'll have to go. My home isn't the place for flare-ups of anger or angst; I'm not unsympathetic and I want to be a good friend, but I can't let my place become a battlefield or a shrink's couch. That's just too much extra stress.

WHAT TO BRING IN

As for bringing home things that are good for you, surround yourself with food, medicines—even clothes, art, and furniture—that are downright good for your health, keep you comfortable and unstressed, or enhance or inspire your life in some way.

There's one item I recommend that satisfies all three of those requirements: plants. Talk about a brilliant technology: Plants are perpetual-motion machines for removing the carbon dioxide that can come from candles, incense, even from your oven—and in my home, that could be a substantial amount of carbon dioxide—and then releasing oxygen back into the room. They reduce dust and pollution and act as a natural air freshener and purifier.

But it isn't just the air that plants improve. Many big companies put plants in their offices because they've actually been shown to increase productivity. Studies have found that office workers suffer less fatigue, fewer dry throats and headaches, even less coughing and skin irritation if there are plants in their environment. Naturally, they work better and harder that way.

Best of all, studies show that people in homes with indoor foliage have reduced stress levels. Maybe it's because plants are beautiful, or because it feels good to take care of a living thing, or because they remind us of the jungles and forests we lived in a zillion years ago. Who cares? Herbs, ferns, flowers: They're good for you. Go get some.

I like to live as green as I can. Not just by having plants—and I have clusters of them all around my place—but by trying to make sure that everything in my home—all the things that surround me—are organic, natural, eco-friendly, healthy, socially conscious, artisanal. . . . You get the picture: I want to be surrounded by things that have been created with care, with thoughtfulness about the planet and its inhabitants.

Yes, you sometimes have to look harder, go farther afield, even pay a bit more for these kinds of products. But there are good reasons to make the extra effort. It isn't just that these things are better for you—and this goes not just for the food you ingest but for everything around you—it's also that by going after such products, you're promoting the people and practices that make them. That's a good feeling to have, as I can testify. And it's why I recommend you try it.

For example, my closet has mostly organically produced clothing items. I love the way they feel on me—thanks to the higher quality of organic fabrics—and I know when I'm wearing them that I'm incorporating sustainability into yet another facet of my life.

Also, I try to fill my home with as many recycled items as possible. I have a knack for finding the sickest vintage trunks and tables at random thrift dives and making them fit, and I favor furniture stores that use recycled or washed-up wood. And here's an added bonus: Sometimes, these kinds of stores are in the more "interesting" or even exotic parts of town—any town, including yours.

To Pump or Not to Pump

There are two ways to administer insulin: through injections or via an insulin pump. Over the past couple of years I have gone back and forth between the two, and each has its advantages.

The pump is like a live-in aide, your own personal Mr. Belvedere. It delivers insulin continuously throughout the day so you experience fewer sudden highs and lows in blood glucose levels. This gives you the freedom to eat more of what you want and when you want it. The injection for the pump is only needed about every 2 or 3 days as opposed to 3 or 4 times a day with the self injections. The pump works best for me when I'm caught up in a busy day, in and out of the kitchen with meetings, etc, and not always able to eat when I should or stick to a schedule. The pump allows me to keep my focus on the task at hand knowing that my insulin intake is being taken care of.

When I am very active, though, I do self-injections. In the summertime, for example, when I'm outside a lot and in and out of the water, I don't want to have to worry about disconnecting vital tubing. Also, without the pump, my load is lighter.

However, there is a certain rogue quality to being off the pump. You have to be more in tune with your body. There's more calculation involved. It's all on you to check and monitor your blood sugar, to recognize when you are getting fatigued, or when a spike or drop happens. When I'm surfing or paddleboarding a long distance, I keep a waterproof box of all my necessities with me: insulin, test kit, syringes, and a snack. That way I'm never caught unprepared if I overdo it. The only real problem with daily injections is that your body can develop resistant areas where you can't absorb insulin properly.

THE KITCHEN

If you want to know what every diabetic should have in the kitchen—in my view, every nondiabetic as well—ask Outkast's Big Boi and André: It's food that's "so fresh and so clean clean." That means greens, grains, fresh fruit, and the highest quality fish and meat—all things natural. You can literally taste the wholesomeness of these foods.

SUSTAINABILITY BEGINS AT HOME

For me, cooking at home is about simplicity. It's about being in my own place taking it all in and doing anything I want just the way I want it. No outside scrutiny, no bloggers, no reviewers or restaurant critics—just me. It's about my energy, and what I feel like cooking and eating at that moment.

Just as important, I try always to be mindful of the concept of sustainability, a phrase that has been widely embraced in foodie circles of late, but that has special resonance to those of us who need to eat carefully and thoughtfully to support our health. First and foremost it means eating only foods that will benefit me, not make my body work overtime to counteract their ill effects. In short, foods that sustain *me* and keep the machine that is my body running full speed ahead. Second, and equally relevant, sustainability means a way of living and eating that doesn't use up everything all at once in a single burst but rather takes advantage of resources while managing to replenish or preserve them. I strive for sustainability in all things, all the time. It can mean taking a stand against the kind of industrial-scale fishing that traps many different species of fish, sea birds, turtles, and marine mammals as "bycatch," then throws those accidental catches back dead or dying into the sea like so much collateral damage. It can mean refusing to buy the veal that's "tenderized" by tying a baby calf to a wall so he can't move his limbs.

For diabetics, though, sustainability has another dimension: Watching what we eat, cooking with care, and just plain being smart about food is our first line of defense against the disease. Eating right, and at the right times, doesn't just provide sustenance, it's literally life-sustaining. So we have an even greater responsibility to make good food choices.

But mostly it means that what I do in the kitchen I do with respect and love for the planet and all its inhabitants—human, animal, even plant. For me in the kitchen, that means finding great ingredients—the freshest and best of the best—seasoning them well but simply, and letting the food speak for itself on the plate.

My way is to start with a really great piece of fresh fish or beautifully butchered meat, season it well—say, with salt, citrus or vinegar, and black pepper—then steam some greens or put together a fresh salad with vine-ripened tomatoes and killer baby greens. Drizzle some great, fruity olive oil over it, sprinkle on some toasted seeds, and top it off with a few drops of grapefruit juice and you have an awesome dish—healthy and fresh, a dish that speaks to everybody, and what it says is: Enjoy the bounty of our planet, respect it, and keep it going.

Keep these ideals in mind—choosing ingredients with care, both for how they are produced and how they will affect your own well-being—and you have the basis for great home cooking.

The recipes in this chapter reflect that. They're all two-handed recipes, which means you can knock them out them easily on your own without tons of prep work and without having to wait too long to sit down and taste them. So they're easy to slap together for one, for a family, or for a dinner party.

Pantry Staples

Here are the staples I stock my pantry with, and monitor almost as stringently as I do the supplies for my health. I recommend them for every kitchen.

- **San Marzano crushed tomatoes**
- **Garlic**
- **Ginger**
- **Chili paste**
- **Soy sauce**
- **Goji berries**
- **Açai**
- **Dried cranberries**

- **Almonds**
- **Cashews**
- **Pickled veggies**
- **Olive oils**
- **Vinegars**
- **Mustards**
- **Quinoa**
- **Almond flour**
- **Agave**
- **Lemons**

There's a great culinary reason these staples are the absolute essentials in my pantry: You can use them with anything, anytime, to create an impromptu, super flavorful, really easy-to-make, and absolutely stellar dish. Add these ingredients to just about anything to change or enhance the flavor or texture or to find new combinations of taste, and I promise you utterly delicious, healthful, beautiful, simple eating.

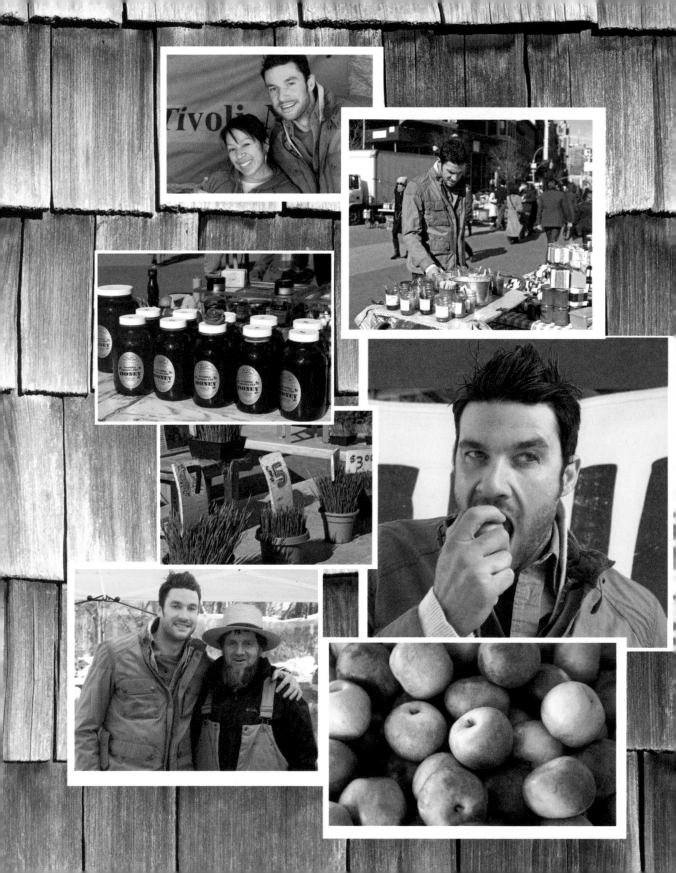

And boy, are they healthy! From lentils to leeks, chicken to cauliflower, beet to bock choy: Pick any dish at all and be assured you're dealing with nutrition heavyweights. I use the word "heavyweights" advisedly. I mean these foods are really fighters. Their fists are right up there protecting you from the debilitating diseases that are making far too many of us frail before our time. They do battle against heart disease. They're full of antioxidants that punch away at the free radicals that can damage your cells. They're packed with vitamins, minerals, and brilliantly colored phytonutrients that can keep a range of cancers at bay.

It's hard for me to express how exciting it is to be a chef who gets to play with foods like this for a living—to start with these beautiful gifts of our planet and create from them finished dishes that nourish the body, give pleasure to the palate, and, in my view, are good for the soul.

You can do the same. In the meantime, play with these recipes—and enjoy the results.

The Artisanal Edge

For more and more chefs these days—as for more and more of the public—sustainable eating isn't just about fish. It's about every type of food we eat, and in this respect, I know we have a lot of company in the general public. So many of you care about this issue of sustainability; it's why the number of natural food stores, greenmarkets, farmstands, and the like are consistently on the rise. And all of this is making it easier for you to do on your own what we do in the haute-cuisine restaurant business. We track down traceable, accountable, artisanal products wherever we can, looking always for the best quality produced in the most eco-friendly manner by farmer, beekeeper, or gardener—because we know that the cream of the crop, the very best products out there, are also the cleanest and the most sustainably produced. That goes for essential finishing essences, or natural oils, that the restaurant orders

handmade by Mandy Aftel from her Aftelier studio in Berkeley, California. It goes for getting the best pork in the world—Ibérico pork from Iberian black pigs farmed in Brooklyn, New York—and the best eggs in the world from Four Story Farms in Pennsylvania.

You can do the same. Google what you're looking for. Check out your local greenmarket or farmstand. Then *ask* for what you want—not just at the greenmarket, but at the supermarket as well. If enough people say they want only the fish that Seafood Watch approves, you can move any market.

Going after these products, identifying them, and finding the right supplier can be something of a challenge, whether you're a professional chef like me or an individual going out to the market, but the effort is worth it. It's just so much better for everyone's health, for the planet we all live on, and for the palate.

Chicken Noodle Soup with Collards and Soul

 6–8

This soup really cures what ails you. I've made it for sick roommates and family members, and I've served it at a Sunday brunch when some people weren't feeling so hot; a few bowls of this and they all felt good again. If you know it's going to be a rainy weekend, and if you and the love of your life plan to duck out of sight for a while, make a pot on Friday night to eat all weekend long. The ginger genuinely warms the soul.

In a large soup pot, heat the oil and butter over medium heat. Throw in the celery, turnips, carrots, onion, garlic, ginger, Old Bay seasoning, paprika, and cumin and cook, stirring constantly, until the onion is translucent and the vegetables have softened, about 3 minutes.

Add the bay leaves and collards and cook for 2 minutes. Stir in the broth, vinegar, hot sauce, and chicken. Cover the pot and bring to a boil. Reduce to a simmer and cook for 50 minutes.

Add the pasta and cook until the pasta is tender, about 10 minutes. Stir in the parsley and season to taste with salt and pepper.

PER SERVING: 175 calories, 11 g protein, 15 g carbohydrates, 8 g total fat (2 g saturated), 24 mg cholesterol, 5 g fiber, 481 mg sodium

- 2 tablespoons olive oil
- 1 tablespoon unsalted butter
- 6 celery ribs, diced
- 2 turnips, peeled and diced
- 2 carrots, diced
- 1 medium onion, diced
- 4 garlic cloves, finely chopped
- ¼ cup finely chopped fresh ginger
- 2 teaspoons Old Bay seasoning
- 1 teaspoon smoked paprika
- 1 teaspoon ground cumin
- 2 bay leaves
- 1 large bunch collard greens, stems and ribs removed, cut into ½-inch-wide ribbons
- 2½ quarts low-sodium chicken broth
- 1 tablespoon white wine vinegar
- 4 dashes hot sauce
- 2 large boneless, skinless chicken thighs, cut into ½-inch pieces
- 1 cup whole wheat pasta bow ties
- ½ cup loosely packed hand-torn flat-leaf parsley
- Salt and freshly ground black pepper

Lentil Broth with Turkey Sausage and Mustard Greens

 I love lentils. My mom made lentils for dinner for us all the time and in my opinion, they're way underappreciated by home cooks. Like beans, lentils are very low on the glycemic index so they won't send your blood sugar spiking through the roof. They're also amazingly energizing; they really keep you going for the long haul. The mustard greens add a much-needed peppery kick to the taste, not to mention a hefty serving of isothiocyanates, sulfur compounds that are thought to fight cancer.

In a large soup pot, heat 2 tablespoons oil over medium-high heat. Add the celery, onions, garlic, ginger, thyme, cinnamon, cumin, and paprika and cook, stirring frequently, until the onions are translucent and the garlic and ginger have softened, 2 to 3 minutes.

Add the lentils, mustard greens, and tomato paste and cook, stirring frequently, for another minute. Add the broth and bring the mixture to a boil. Reduce to a simmer and cook, uncovered, until the lentils are tender, about 1 hour 15 minutes.

Meanwhile, in a medium skillet, cook the sausage over medium-high until browned, 4 to 5 minutes.

Once the lentils have finished cooking, add the browned sausage to the pot, along with the vinegar and a splash of olive oil. Season to taste with salt and pepper.

Spoon the lentils into 8 individual soup bowls and top each serving with 1 tablespoon of the Parmesan.

PER SERVING: 230 calories, 15 g protein, 24 g carbohydrates, 9 g total fat (1 g saturated), 19 mg cholesterol, 7 g fiber, 741 mg sodium

- 2 **tablespoons extra-virgin olive oil, plus more for finishing**
- 1 **bunch celery, finely diced**
- 2 **small yellow onions, finely diced**
- 4 **garlic cloves, smashed and finely chopped**
- 2 **tablespoons finely chopped fresh ginger**
- 2 **tablespoons fresh thyme leaves**
- 1 **teaspoon ground cinnamon**
- 1 **teaspoon ground cumin**
- 1 **teaspoon smoked paprika**
- ½ **pound green lentils**
- 1 **large bunch mustard greens, stems and center ribs discarded, leaves coarsely chopped**
- 2 **tablespoons tomato paste**
- 2 **quarts low-sodium chicken broth**
- ½ **pound turkey sausage, casings removed, cut into ¼-inch-thick chunks**
- 2 **tablespoons red wine vinegar**
  Salt and freshly ground black pepper
- 4 **tablespoons shaved Parmesan cheese**

clam chowder

 People swear by their chowder. They might bet their firstborn that it's the best. Well, here's another to throw in the recipe basket, and this one obviously has some twists and turns that are a bit different. Why, you ask? I made this for the lovers of this classic soup who hate the bottomless calories and fat of yesteryear's clam chowda. It has all the classic components, but I've tweaked them in a necessary way to get the final product that we're looking for. I think you're really going to like this one—hopefully better than the ones you're accustomed to.

In a medium saucepan, heat the oil over medium-high heat. Add the bacon and cook until the fat is rendered and the bacon begins to brown, 2 to 3 minutes. Add the potatoes, onion, celery, garlic, Old Bay seasoning, and celery seeds. Cook, stirring frequently, until the onion and celery are translucent, 2 to 3 minutes.

Sprinkle the rice flour over the vegetables and stir for 1 minute to make a roux. Add the canned minced clams and wine, stirring well to combine. Pour in the clam juice, broth, milk, Worcestershire sauce, and hot sauce. Bring the soup to a simmer and cook, stirring occasionally, until the potatoes are fork-tender, about 45 minutes.

Add the whole clams and the dill, cover the pot and cook until the clams open, 8 to 10 minutes. Discard any unopened shells. Season to taste with salt and pepper.

PER SERVING: 236 calories, 15 g protein, 25 g carbohydrates, 7 g total fat (1 g saturated), 32 mg cholesterol, 3 g fiber, 1,169 mg sodium

- 2 tablespoons olive oil
- 2 slices thick-cut bacon, chopped into small pieces
- 1 pound red or white russet potatoes, peeled and coarsely chopped
- 1 large Vidalia or yellow onion, diced
- 2 celery ribs, diced
- 2 garlic cloves, finely chopped
- 1½ teaspoons Old Bay seasoning
- 1 tablespoon celery seeds
- ¼ cup rice flour
- 2 8 ounce cans minced clams
- ½ cup dry white wine
- 2 cups bottled clam juice
- 2 cups low-sodium chicken broth
- 1 cup almond milk
- 1 tablespoon Worcestershire sauce
- 1 tablespoon hot sauce
- 2 dozen Little Neck clams, scrubbed
- ½ cup chopped fresh dill
- Salt and freshly ground black pepper

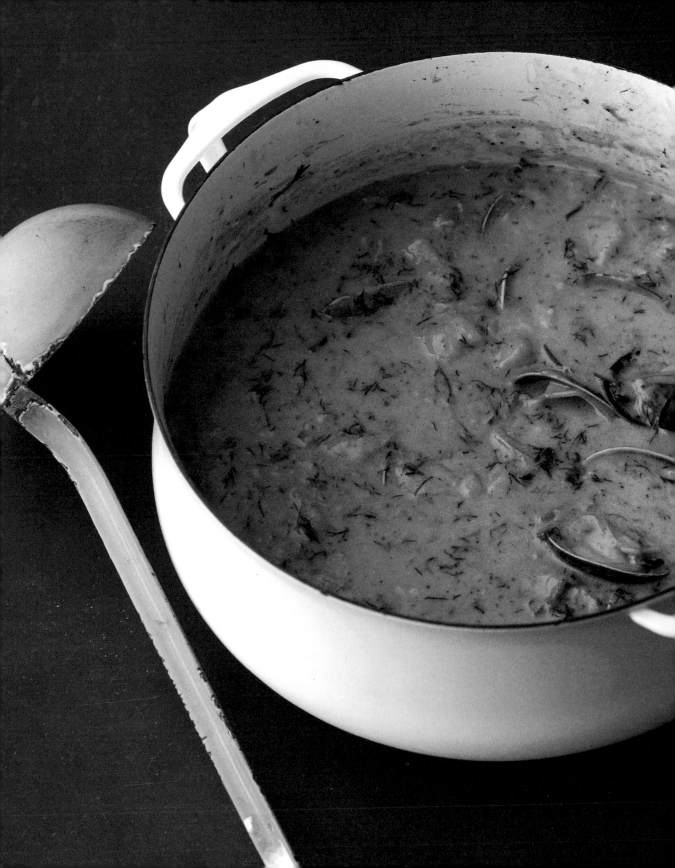

Lemon–Basil Roast Chicken

 Everyone needs a solid recipe for a roast chicken. Everyone. It's an American classic, and when done right, it's aces—versatile, flavorful, and moist. Plus, it's packed with protein and cancer-preventing niacin. So go!

Preheat the oven to 350°F. Discard the chicken giblets. Rinse the chicken and pat it dry. Place the chicken in a roasting pan and season it liberally with salt and pepper, inside and out.

In a small bowl, mix together the butter, oil, agave nectar, lemon zest and juice, garlic, basil, thyme, 1 teaspoon salt, and ½ teaspoon pepper. Rub the mixture all over the chicken and season the chicken once more with a couple dashes of salt and pepper. Stuff the chicken's cavity with any excess seasoning and the 2 used lemons.

Transfer the chicken to the oven and roast until a meat thermometer inserted in the thickest part of the thigh (without touching bone) registers 180°F, about 1 hour 45 minutes. Remove the chicken from the oven and let it rest for 5 minutes before carving.

PER SERVING: 224 calories, 24 g protein, 6 g carbohydrates, 12 g total fat (4 g saturated), 86 mg cholesterol, 1 g fiber, 473 mg sodium

1 whole free-range organic chicken (3 pounds)

Salt and freshly ground black pepper

2 tablespoons unsalted butter, at room temperature

2 tablespoons olive oil

1 tablespoon agave nectar

Grated zest and juice of 2 lemons

4 cloves garlic, smashed and finely chopped

1 cup thinly sliced fresh basil leaves

Leaves from 1 bunch of fresh thyme

Roasted Chicken with Cauliflower and Broccoli and Mustard Vinaigrette

 When we need something fast that the staff at Surf Lodge can get down before service starts, Brittney and Jasa often throw this together. With its crispy brown skin and robust flavor, this roasted chicken is a healthier alternative to fried chicken, and the cauliflower-broccoli sauté is packed with tons of essential nutrients and vitamins. I ask the girls to make me this dish a *lot*.

To marinate the chicken: In a large bowl, mix together the lemon zest and juice, parsley, garlic powder, onion powder, coriander, and 4 tablespoons of the oil. Add the chicken, turning to coat in the marinade. Cover the bowl tightly with plastic wrap and refrigerate for at least 2 hours or overnight.

Preheat the oven to 400°F. Remove the chicken from the marinade and season liberally with salt and pepper. In a large oven-proof skillet, heat 1 tablespoon of oil over high heat until very hot. Add the chicken and sear for 2 minutes on each side.

Transfer the skillet to the oven and roast skin-side up until the chicken is golden brown and a thermometer inserted in the thickest portion registers 160°F, about 15 minutes.

Meanwhile, to cook the vegetables: In a large skillet, heat 2 tablespoons of the oil over medium-low heat. Add the shallots and garlic and cook until the garlic is soft and the shallots are translucent, 2 to 3 minutes. Toss in the cauliflower and broccoli and cook, stirring frequently, until the florets are fork-tender, 2 to 3 minutes. Season to taste with salt and pepper.

To make the mustard vinaigrette: Heat a medium skillet over medium-high heat. Add the garlic and toast until lightly browned, about 2 minutes. Transfer the toasted garlic to a small bowl and whisk in the lemon juice, mustard, oil, agave nectar, shallots, and thyme.

Drizzle the vinaigrette over the finished chicken breasts and serve with the cauliflower-broccoli sauté.

PER SERVING: 608 calories, 41 g protein, 19 g carbohydrates, 41 g total fat (8 g saturated), 116 mg cholesterol, 3 g fiber, 415 mg sodium

Grated zest and juice of 2 lemons

1 tablespoon chopped flat-leaf parsley

2 teaspoons garlic powder

2 teaspoons onion powder

2 teaspoons ground coriander

7 tablespoons olive oil

4 bone-in, skin-on chicken breast halves (8 to 10 ounces each)

Salt and freshly ground black pepper

3 tablespoons chopped shallots

3 tablespoons chopped garlic

2 cups cauliflower florets

2 cups broccoli florets

MUSTARD VINAIGRETTE

1 tablespoon chopped garlic

Juice of 2 lemons

3 tablespoons Dijon mustard

2 tablespoons extra-virgin olive oil

1 tablespoon agave nectar

1 tablespoon chopped shallots

1 tablespoon chopped fresh thyme leaves

Pulled Blackened Chicken with Toasted Couscous

 Manna, a 24-hour Middle Eastern/Mediterranean restaurant that is just down the street from my apartment in Williamsburg, Brooklyn, makes great traditional dishes like okra hummus and stuffed grape leaves—but my favorite by far is their roasted chicken with turmeric-scented couscous. It's a dish that should be on everyone's weeknight to-do list.

To roast the chicken: Preheat the oven to 350°F. Remove the chicken giblets. Rinse the chicken and pat it dry.

In a small bowl, toss together the garlic, blackening seasoning, oil, lemon halves, thyme sprigs, salt, and pepper. Remove the lemon and thyme from the seasoning mixture and stick them into the cavity of the chicken. Rub the seasoning mixture all over the chicken and transfer the bird to a roasting pan.

Roast the chicken until a thermometer inserted in the thickest part of the thigh registers 180°F, 45 to 50 minutes. Remove the chicken from the oven, take the lemon halves out of the cavity, and squeeze them over the chicken. Let the chicken cool for 10 minutes, then, pull the meat off in chunks.

Meanwhile, to make the couscous: In a medium saucepan, combine the almond milk and broth and bring to a rolling simmer over medium-high heat; keep on a back burner.

In another medium saucepan, heat the oil over medium-high heat. Add the onion, garlic, pine nuts, cinnamon, and turmeric. Cook until the spices bloom and the aromatics take over the room, about 2 minutes. Add the couscous and cook, stirring, until it is golden brown, 2 to 3 minutes.

Transfer the couscous to a large bowl and pour in the hot milk-broth mixture. Add the scallions. Cover the bowl tightly with plastic wrap and steam for at least 20 minutes.

Season the couscous liberally with salt and pepper, then sprinkle with the lemon juice. Stir in the pulled chicken shreds to combine and serve warm.

PER SERVING: 613 calories, 33 g protein, 28 g carbohydrates, 41 g total fat (8 g saturated), 110 mg cholesterol, 3 g fiber, 724 mg sodium

BLACKENED CHICKEN

- 1 3-pound free-range organic chicken
- 4 garlic cloves, finely chopped
- ¼ cup blackening seasoning
- 2 tablespoons olive oil
- 1 lemon, halved
- ½ bunch fresh thyme
- 1 teaspoon fine sea salt
- ½ teaspoon freshly ground black pepper

TOASTED COUSCOUS

- 1½ cups almond milk
- ½ cup reduced-sodium chicken broth
- 3 tablespoons olive oil
- 1 large onion, finely diced
- 4 garlic cloves, finely chopped
- ½ cup pine nuts
- 1 teaspoon ground cinnamon
- 1 teaspoon turmeric
- 1 cup Israeli couscous
- 2 scallions, thinly sliced
- Salt and freshly ground black pepper
- Juice of 2 lemons

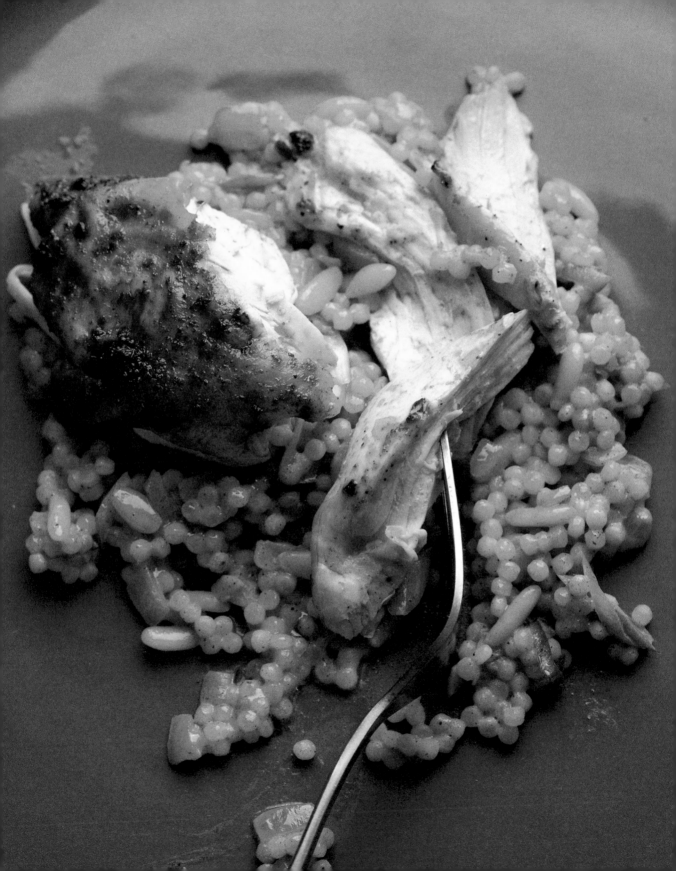

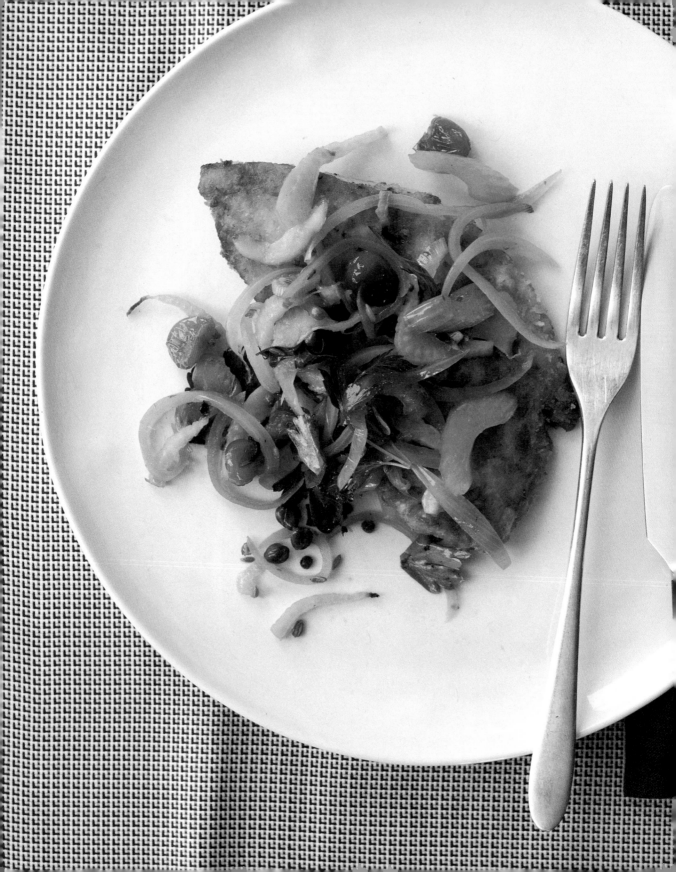

Turkey Paillards with Cranberry Piccata Sauce

 Chicken paillards—boneless breast fillets pounded to an even thickness—are a huge staple in New York City restaurants. Every bistro in town has them, and between the hours of noon and 1:30 p.m. everyone in a suit—man or woman—can be found scarfing one down, usually served over a handful of arugula for a boring, effortless salad. I start with a roasted turkey breast so it has to stay in the pan only long enough to crisp and brown the breading, making this a perfect quick weeknight dinner. Trust me, once you go turkey, you'll never go back.

To make the sauce: Preheat the oven to 450°F. Spread the fennel on a baking sheet, drizzle with 1 tablespoon of the olive oil, and bake until browned on the edges, about 6 minutes. Set aside to cool to room temperature.

In a large skillet, heat the remaining 2 tablespoons olive oil over medium-high heat. Add the onions, celery, and fennel seeds and cook until the onions and celery are translucent, about 2 minutes. Add the white wine cook for 2 minutes, stirring with a wooden spoon to scrape up any browned bits from the bottom of the pan to deglaze it. Add the toasted fennel, cranberries, parsley, capers, sweetener, pink pepper, and butter and cook for 2 to 3 minutes to heat through. Remove the pan from the heat.

To cook the paillards: In a shallow bowl, whisk together the milk and eggs to make an egg wash. In another shallow bowl, combine the panko, flour, and Parmesan. Dip each piece of turkey in the egg wash, coating both sides, then dip into the breading mixture. Shake off any excess breading.

In a large skillet, heat the canola oil over medium-high heat. Add the turkey and pan-fry until golden brown, 2 to 3 minutes on each side.

Serve each paillard topped with ¼ cup of the cranberry piccata sauce. You will have leftovers for another meal.

PER SERVING: 496 calories, 51 g protein, 14 g carbohydrates, 24 g total fat (6 g saturated), 218 mg cholesterol, 3 g fiber, 303 mg sodium

CRANBERRY PICCATA SAUCE

- 1 medium fennel bulb (about ¾ pound), stalks discarded, cored, and thinly sliced
- 3 tablespoons olive oil
- 1 small yellow onion, diced
- ½ bunch celery, thinly sliced
- 1½ teaspoons fennel seeds
- ½ cup dry white wine
- 1 cup fresh cranberries
- ¼ cup hand-torn flat-leaf parsley
- 1 tablespoon drained capers
- 1 to 2 tablespoons stevia extract
- 1½ teaspoons freshly ground pink peppercorns
- 2 tablespoons unsalted butter

TURKEY PAILLARDS

- ½ cup whole milk
- 2 cage-free organic eggs
- ½ cup panko breadcrumbs
- ½ cup almond flour
- ¼ cup grated Parmesan cheese
- 4 thick slices (6 ounces each) fully cooked turkey breast
- 2 tablespoons canola oil

Steamed Marinated Chicken with Serious Bok Choy

 When I'm so crazy busy I don't even have time to scramble myself an egg for dinner, my quick and easy fallback is ordering steamed chicken and broccoli from the take-out place down the street. During one particularly rough patch I realized I was doing this 2 or 3 times a week—and then I realized how much money I was spending having someone else do the cooking! So I started planning ahead, putting the chicken in the fridge to marinate when I had a few minutes, and then throwing everything into the steamer when hunger pangs hit. And guess what? It is faster, fresher, and way better—not to mention cheaper. It took way too long to realize this, but better late than never.

Place the chicken in a large bowl. Add the sesame oil, rice wine, soy sauce, lime and lemon juices, ginger, garlic, and cilantro and toss well to combine. Cover the bowl tightly with plastic wrap and refrigerate for at least 1 hour or overnight.

Add 2 inches of water to a wok or large saucepan and set a bamboo steamer in the pan, making sure the bottom of the steamer is just above, not touching, the water level. Line the bottom of the steamer with the cabbage leaves. Cover, bring the water to a boil over medium-high heat, add the marinated chicken, and steam until the chicken is cooked through, 10 to 12 minutes.

Meanwhile, in a medium skillet, heat the garlic oil over medium-high heat. Add the onion and sambal and cook until the onions are translucent, 2 to 3 minutes. Add the bok choy and cook, stirring frequently, until it is fork-tender, 5 to 6 minutes.

Serve the chicken over the bok choy and season to taste with salt and pepper.

PER SERVING: 397 calories, 40 g protein, 16 g carbohydrates, 20 g total fat (3 g saturated), 110 mg cholesterol, 3 g fiber, 764 mg sodium

1½ **pounds boneless, skinless free-range organic chicken breasts, cut into 1-inch pieces**

2 **tablespoons toasted sesame oil**

2 **tablespoons rice wine**

2 **tablespoons reduced-sodium soy sauce**

Juice of 2 limes

Juice of 2 lemons

2 **tablespoons finely chopped fresh ginger**

2 **tablespoons smashed and chopped garlic**

¼ **cup chopped fresh cilantro**

4 **cabbage or lettuce leaves**

2 **tablespoons Roasted Garlic Oil (page 93)**

1 **large onion, finely diced**

1 **tablespoon sambal oelek chili paste**

1 **head bok choy (about 1 pound), cut crosswise into 1-inch-wide slices**

Salt and freshly ground black pepper

Baby Greens with Lemon, Ginger, and Crispy Pork

(4)

I love Chinese food—not the typical take-out kind that's loaded with MSG and slathered with corn syrup, but authentic, genuine, real-deal Chinese food. In Chinese cuisine, the ancestry and the pride go back thousands of years. When I look for the really worthy cooks of this incredible cuisine, I think about the elderly women of the community, the ones who've been perfecting this cuisine every day of their lives—just doing it and doing it well. No fuss, no crap—just real, good food.

In a medium skillet, heat the oil over medium heat. Add the bacon and cook just until it starts to crackle and turn golden brown, 2 to 3 minutes. Add the onion, garlic, ginger, lemongrass, and fennel seeds to the pan and cook for 2 to 3 minutes, or until the onion is translucent.

Remove the pan from the heat and pour off all but 1 tablespoon of fat. Set the bacon mixture aside to cool to room temperature.

In a large bowl, combine the baby greens, mâche, cilantro, arugula, radishes, and lemon zest and juice. Drizzle with the cider vinegar and rice vinegar and give the salad a gentle toss until thoroughly combined.

Once the bacon mixture has reached room temperature, chop the bacon and add it to the bowl. Scrape the sautéed onion mixture and the fat from the skillet into the bowl. Toss well, season to taste with salt and pepper, and serve to a greedy crowd.

PER SERVING: 243 calories, 11 g protein, 9 g carbohydrates, 19 g total fat (5 g saturated), 24 mg cholesterol, 2 g fiber, 608 mg sodium

2 tablespoons olive oil

¼ pound thick-cut smoked bacon

1 large yellow onion, thinly sliced

3 garlic cloves, smashed and finely chopped

2 tablespoons finely chopped fresh ginger

1 tablespoon finely chopped fresh lemongrass

1 tablespoon fennel seeds

2 cups mixed baby greens

1 cup mâche

½ cup loosely packed fresh cilantro

½ cup loosely packed baby arugula

2 radishes, shaved on a mandoline or sliced into paper-thin discs

Grated zest and juice of 1 lemon

1 tablespoon cider vinegar

1 tablespoon rice vinegar

Salt and freshly ground black pepper

Seared Strip Loin with Ginger and Chives

 Here's a great example of why I am so hooked on ginger in action. These are the steaks you want to come home to. Get yourself a bottle of the best, and don't make any after-dinner plans.

In a large bowl, whisk together 3 tablespoons of the garlic oil, 3 tablespoons of the chives, 2 tablespoons of the ginger, the chopped garlic, shallot, tamari, and vinegar. Add the steaks to the marinade, cover the bowl with plastic wrap, and set aside to marinate at room temperature for 30 minutes.

In a large skillet, heat the butter and the remaining 2 tablespoons garlic oil over high heat. Remove the steaks from the marinade and season generously with salt and pepper. Add the steaks to the pan and sear for 2 minutes on each side, until they are golden brown and medium-rare. On the final turn of the steaks, add the remaining 1 tablespoon chives and 1 tablespoon ginger to the pan. Spoon the pan juices, ginger, and chives from the pan over the steaks as they cook for their final minute.

Transfer the steaks to a cutting board and let them rest for 5 minutes before slicing against the grain.

5 tablespoons Roasted Garlic Oil (page 93)

4 tablespoons chopped fresh chives

3 tablespoons finely chopped fresh ginger

4 garlic cloves, smashed and finely chopped

1 shallot, finely diced

2 tablespoons tamari

2 tablespoons red wine vinegar

2 strip loin steaks (12 to 14 ounces each), preferably aged

1 tablespoon unsalted butter

Salt and freshly ground black pepper

PER SERVING: 461 calories, 39 g protein, 5 g carbohydrates, 31 g total fat (8 g saturated), 102 mg cholesterol, 0.5 g fiber, 102 mg sodium

Sicilian Cauliflower with Anchovies

 My grandfather, a man I try to emulate on a daily basis, was Sicilian, and this dish is for him. He didn't cook—he was a fireman, actually—but he was a great guy and a great family man. My mom adored her father, as daughters tend to do. I have made many versions of this dish; I even prepared one on *Top Chef*.

Bring a large pot of generously salted water to a boil over high heat. Add the cauliflower and cook for 30 seconds. Drain into a colander and run the florets under cold water for 1 minute to stop the cooking. Transfer the florets to a large bowl. Add the vinegar, olive oil, garlic oil, olives, gherkins, anchovies, capers, parsley, pepper flakes, and the chopped eggs. Toss the mixture gently and season to taste with salt and pepper.

Cover the bowl with plastic wrap and refrigerate for at least 2 hours before serving.

PER SERVING: 168 calories, 8 g protein, 5 g carbohydrates, 13 g total fat (3 g saturated), 166 mg cholesterol, 2 g fiber, 645 mg sodium

- 2 **cups bite-sized cauliflower florets**
- 2 **tablespoons red wine vinegar**
- 1 **tablespoon olive oil**
- 1 **tablespoon Roasted Garlic Oil (page 93)**
- ¼ **cup finely chopped kalamata olives**
- ¼ **cup finely chopped green olives**
- ¼ **cup finely chopped gherkins (baby pickles)**
- 8 **oil-packed anchovy fillets— drained, smashed with the back of a knife, and finely chopped**
- 2 **tablespoons drained and chopped capers**
- ¼ **cup thinly sliced flat-leaf parsley leaves**
- 1 **teaspoon red pepper flakes**
- 3 **hard boiled eggs, chopped**
- **Sea salt and freshly ground black pepper**

Spiced Brussels Sprouts with Cider Vinegar

Funny how life comes full circle. I vividly remember sitting at my mom's dinner table at 11215 Provincetown Lane screaming about eating those horrible little green balls handed to us by Lucifer himself. I mean at least that's what you would've thought if you saw me carrying on about how much I downright loathed them. (Sadly, I wasn't a 4-year-old having temper tantrums; I was closer to 16.) Now, though, I love them. Broiled, sautéed, roasted, fried—don't care, I'd eat them all day every day. With the right amount of acid-to-fat content, these sprouts are right on time. Season well and forget the thoughts of Lucifer; focus on the fact that they are high in fiber, B vitamins, and cancer-fighting sulfur compounds.

In a large skillet, heat the oil over medium-high heat. Add the shallot, ginger, cumin, turmeric, cinnamon, fennel seeds, and chili paste and cook, stirring frequently, until the shallots are translucent, 2 to 3 minutes.

Add the Brussels sprouts, toss well to combine, and cook until they are fork-tender, about 3 minutes.

Stir in the vinegar, broth, agave nectar, parsley, and sesame seeds and cook for 2 minutes to heat through. Season to taste with salt and pepper.

PER SERVING: 158 calories, 3 g protein, 15 g carbohydrates, 11 g total fat (1 g saturated), 22 mg cholesterol, 3 g fiber, 44 mg sodium

¼ cup Roasted Garlic Oil (page 93)

1 shallot, finely diced

2 tablespoons finely chopped fresh ginger

1 tablespoon ground cumin

1½ teaspoons turmeric

1 teaspoon ground cinnamon

1 teaspoon fennel seeds

½ teaspoon chili paste

1 pound Brussels sprouts, trimmed and quartered

3 tablespoons cider vinegar

3 tablespoons reduced-sodium chicken broth

2 tablespoons agave nectar

½ cup loosely packed hand-torn flat-leaf parsley

1 tablespoon sesame seeds

Salt and freshly ground black pepper

Braised Leeks with Kalamata Olives, Tomatoes, and Basil

 Leeks are something of a culinary underdog that get a lot less press than, say, Vidalia onions. Don't overlook these babies, because they are brilliant grilled, broiled, charred, baked, or braised. Just make sure you wash 'em well under cold running water because they can harbor a lot of sand or grit.

Preheat the oven to 400°F.

Trim the roots and any dark wilted tops of the leeks; pull off any damaged outer leaves. Halve the leeks lengthwise. Rinse the leek halves thoroughly in cold water (making sure to get the hidden grit at the spot where the light colored portion starts to turn a darker green). Pat them dry.

Heat a large skillet over medium-high heat and add the roasted garlic oil. Working in batches, add the leeks, cut-side down, and sear for 3 to 4 minutes. Season the leeks with salt and pepper, then turn to cook on the other side for 1 minute. Transfer the leeks to a Dutch oven or a baking dish with a tight-fitting lid.

Add the shallots to the skillet and cook over medium-high heat until aromatic, 2 to 3 minutes. Add ¼ cup water, the broth, tomatoes, olives, thyme, lemon juice, and honey. Bring the mixture to a boil, then remove from the heat and pour it over the leeks. Be careful not to completely cover the leeks with the liquid.

Cover the leeks, transfer to the oven, and braise until the leeks are fork-tender, about 35 minutes. Gently stir in the basil and serve hot.

6 large leeks

¼ cup Roasted Garlic Oil (page 93)

Salt and freshly ground black pepper

2 shallots, finely diced

2 cups reduced-sodium chicken broth

1½ cups canned crushed San Marzano tomatoes

¼ cup chopped kalamata olives

2 tablespoons chopped fresh thyme leaves

Juice of 1 lemon

1 tablespoon orange blossom honey

½ cup loosely packed hand-torn fresh basil

PER SERVING: 181 calories, 3 g protein, 21 g carbohydrates, 10 g total fat (2 g saturated), 0 mg cholesterol, 3 g fiber, 359 mg sodium

Zucchini Pancakes

 This is a dish that rocks any time of year. It can easily become a favorite for summer picnics and Sunday brunches, and if you make this dish for your mother, you'll become her favorite. It's just that good, and it's easy—I promise.

Wrap the grated zucchini in a clean kitchen towel and twist the towel to wring out as much liquid as possible.

In a large bowl, mix together the zucchini, ginger, lemon zest, agave nectar, and eggs. Add the flour, baking powder, salt, and pepper and mix until combined.

In a large nonstick skillet, heat the oil over medium-high heat. Once the oil begins to shimmer, reduce the heat to medium-low. Working in batches, drop a large spoonful of batter per pancake into the pan. Cook the pancakes until golden brown, about 2 minutes per side. Serve hot.

PER SERVING: 98 calories, 5 g protein, 12 g carbohydrates, 4 g total fat (1 g saturated), 108 mg cholesterol, 2 g fiber, 520 mg sodium

1 **pound zucchini, coarsely grated (about 4 cups)**

1 **tablespoon coarsely grated fresh ginger**

1 **tablespoon grated lemon zest**

1 **tablespoon agave nectar**

3 **cage-free organic eggs, lightly beaten**

⅓ **cup whole wheat flour**

1 **tablespoon baking powder**

1 **teaspoon fine sea salt**

1 **teaspoon freshly ground black pepper**

1½ **teaspoons olive oil**

Cucumber, Mint, and Yuzu Salad

6

I love superfast, easy salads that you can just whip or sling into gear with no skill required and no effort whatsoever. When you're on the go, always running around, and you finally get a chance to cook for yourself, the last thing you really want to do is cook for yourself. So having simple recipes like this on hand can be crucial for your lifestyle. They are for mine.

In a large bowl, combine the cucumbers, bean sprouts, mint, yuzu juice, agave nectar, chili powder, and 2 tablespoons of the oil. Toss well and set aside.

In a medium skillet, heat the remaining 2 tablespoons of oil over medium-high heat. Add the garlic, ginger, and onion, and cook until the onion is translucent and the garlic and ginger have softened, 2 to 3 minutes. Set aside to cool to room temperature.

Add the onion mixture to the cucumber mixture and season to taste with salt and pepper. Toss well to combine.

PER SERVING: 106 calories, 1 g protein, 6 g carbohydrates, 9 g total fat (1 g saturated), 0 mg cholesterol, 1 g fiber, 2 mg sodium

- 2 **hothouse cucumbers, quartered lengthwise, then sliced crosswise**
- 1 **handful bean sprouts**
- ¼ **cup chopped fresh mint leaves**
- ¼ **cup yuzu juice**
- 1 **tablespoon agave nectar**
- 1 **teaspoon chili powder**
- ¼ **cup Roasted Garlic Oil (on this page)**
- 2 **tablespoons smashed and finely chopped garlic**
- 2 **tablespoons finely chopped fresh ginger**
- 2 **tablespoons diced yellow onion**

  Salt and freshly ground black pepper

Roasted Garlic and Roasted Garlic Oil

Roasted garlic adds a rich dimension to so many different dishes—and it's super easy to prepare. I usually roast about 2 heads of garlic at a time, but this recipe is easily halved.

In a large saucepan, heat the oil over low heat. Once the oil begins to shimmer (be careful not to let it boil), add the garlic cloves. Cook the garlic uncovered for 1 hour and 15 minutes, or until the cloves are easily mashed with a fork. Store the cooled oil and garlic cloves in a covered container in the refrigerator for up to 2 weeks.

- 2 **cups grapeseed oil**
- 20 **garlic cloves (about 2 heads), peeled**

Sautéed Squash with Olive Oil, Toasted Pumpkin Seeds, and Pecorino

 I love eating at Mario Batali's pizza restaurant, Otto, especially in the fall when the air is a bit nippy. It has a homey and beautiful bar that's a good spot for a late-afternoon glass of wine. It always has six to eight very rustic, simple, and seasonal vegetable preparations, one of which inspired this unassuming and subtle squash dish. This version is made with yellow summer squash, but you can also use winter squash and the seeds other times of the year, adjusting the cooking time as necessary.

In a medium skillet, heat the oil over medium-high heat. Add the garlic, shallot, and pumpkin seeds and cook until the pumpkin seeds are toasted and the garlic and onions are translucent, 2 to 3 minutes. Add the squash and cook, stirring frequently, until the squash is golden brown and fork tender, 4 to 6 minutes.

Toss in the parsley and chives and season well with salt and pepper. Top each serving with a sprinkle of pecorino cheese.

PER SERVING: 229 calories, 9 g protein, 9 g carbohydrates, 18 g total fat (3 g saturated), 2 mg cholesterol, 3 g fiber, 193 mg sodium

2 tablespoons olive oil

2 garlic cloves, smashed and finely chopped

1 shallot, finely chopped

½ cup raw pumpkin seeds (pepitas)

2 large yellow squash, cut into ¼-inch-thick half-moons

¼ cup thinly sliced flat-leaf parsley

2 tablespoons finely chopped fresh chives

Salt and freshly ground black pepper

2 tablespoons finely grated pecorino cheese

Broccoli with Citrus and Garlic Oil

This dish doesn't cure diabetes—nothing does—but it can control the damage diabetes inflicts on the blood vessels of the heart. This is probably due to a substance called sulforaphane found in all cruciferous vegetables and in its highest concentration in broccoli. That's why I try to eat broccoli every day—though I can't say I am 100 percent successful in that goal. It is really so damn good for you you'd be crazy not to eat this stuff all the time. I either make it spicy or give it a lot of citrus. Or both, as in this recipe. Get some.

In a large skillet, heat the oil over medium heat. Add the onion and garlic and cook, stirring frequently, until the onion is translucent, 2 to 3 minutes. Toss in the broccoli and red pepper flakes and cook until the broccoli is bright green, 1 to 2 minutes. Add the wine, broth, orange zest and juice, and lemon zest and juice and cook for about 2 minutes to incorporate the flavors. Season to taste with salt and black pepper.

PER SERVING: 143 calories, 2 g protein, 11 g carbohydrates, 11 g total fat (2 g saturated), 0 mg cholesterol, 2 g fiber, 237 mg sodium

- 3 **tablespoons Roasted Garlic Oil (page 93)**
- ½ **Vidalia or other sweet onion, thinly sliced**
- 3 **garlic cloves, smashed and finely chopped**
- 2 **cups bite-size broccoli florets**
- ½ **teaspoon red pepper flakes**
- ½ **cup dry white wine**
- ½ **cup low-sodium chicken broth**
- **Grated zest and juice of 1 orange**
- **Grated zest and juice of 1 lemon**
- **Salt and freshly ground black pepper**

Roasted Beets with Ginger and Bacon

 Beets are just simply delicious, and few foods are more gorgeous on the plate. The ginger adds real depth to the dish as well as imparts aromatic niceties. Omit the smoky bacon if you like, but it does cut the sweetness of the beets nicely. Make this a side dish or a whole meal; I do both.

Preheat the oven to 450°F. Place the beets and rosemary in the center of a large piece of foil. Drizzle 2 tablespoons of the oil over them and season generously with salt and pepper. Fold up the edges of the foil to make a bowl shape. Transfer the packet to a baking sheet and roast until they are easily pierced with the tip of a knife, about 1 hour. When the beets are cool enough to handle, use a clean kitchen towel to rub off the skins. Then cut the beets into ½-inch cubes.

Meanwhile, in a large skillet, heat the remaining 3 tablespoons oil over medium-high heat. Add the bacon and cook, stirring frequently, until the bacon begins to brown, 2 to 3 minutes. Add the onion, fennel, garlic, ginger, agave nectar, and mustard. Cook until the onion is translucent and the fennel has softened, 2 to 3 minutes.

Carefully drain the fat out of the skillet and discard. Stir the vinegar and parsley into the bacon mixture and season to taste with salt and pepper. Transfer the mixture to a large bowl.

Add the beets to the bowl with the bacon mixture. Toss well to combine.

To serve, spread the watercress leaves on a serving platter, sprinkle with the lemon zest and juice, and top with the beet mixture.

PER SERVING: 368 calories, 16 g protein, 18 g carbohydrates, 28 g total fat (6 g saturated), 63 mg cholesterol, 4 g fiber, 934 mg sodium

1 **pound beets, trimmed and scrubbed**

3 **sprigs rosemary**

5 **tablespoons extra-virgin olive oil**

Salt and freshly ground black pepper

½ **pound thick-cut smoked bacon, chopped**

1 **large yellow onion, diced**

1 **large fennel bulb (about 1 pound), stalks discarded, cored, and finely chopped**

4 **garlic cloves, smashed and finely chopped**

¼ **cup finely chopped fresh ginger**

1 **tablespoon agave nectar**

1 **tablespoon Dijon mustard**

2 **tablespoons cider vinegar**

¼ **cup chopped flat-leaf parsley**

1 **bunch (about ½ pound) watercress, tough stems removed**

Grated zest and juice of 2 lemons

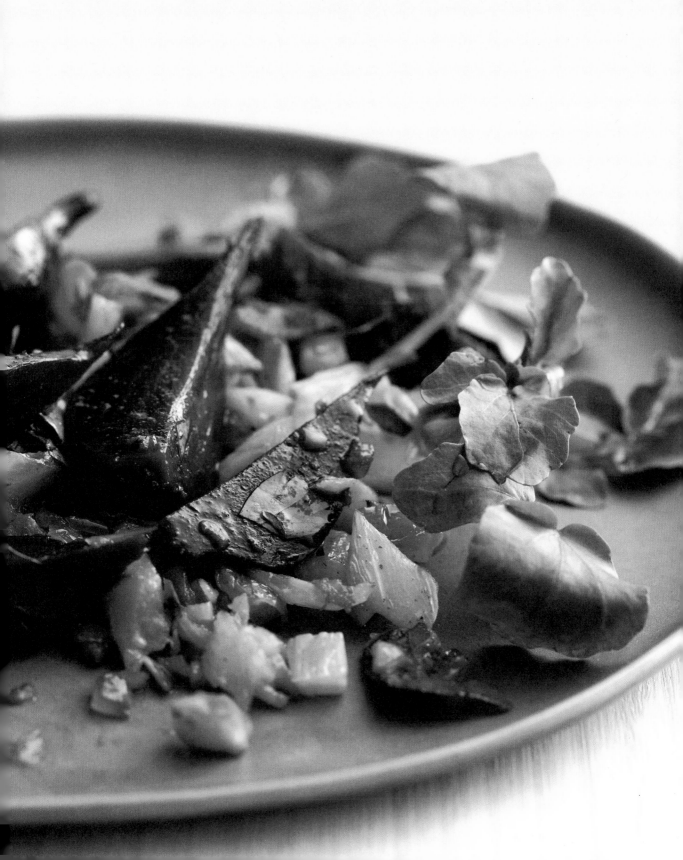

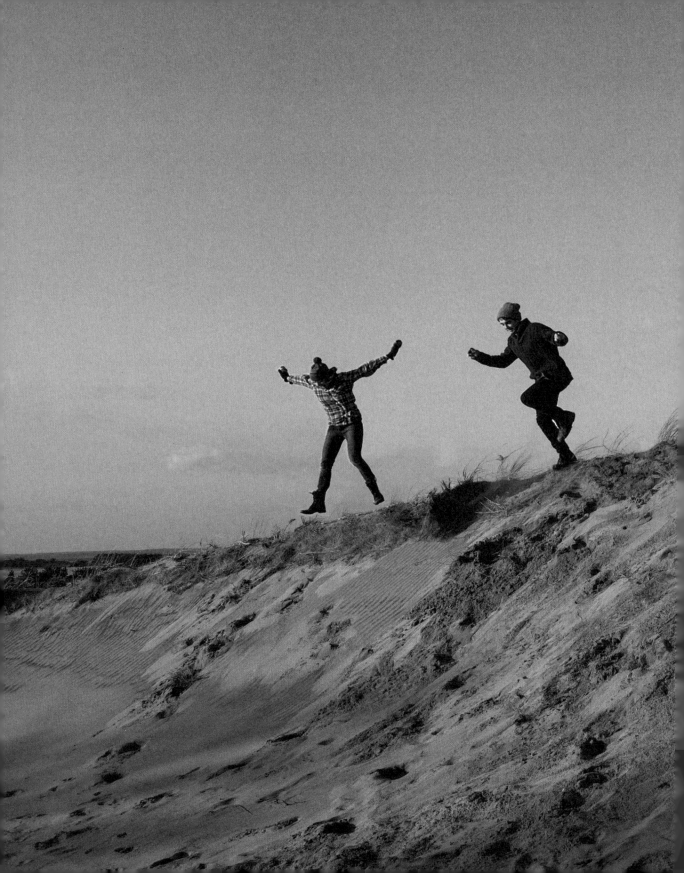

Chapter Four

STAYING
ENERGIZED

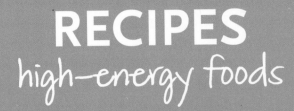

RECIPES
high-energy foods

The Sweet Life is a high-energy life that demands high-energy food. But it also needs motion, exercise, a conscious effort to keep our bodies fit and strong and nimble—because the more we do, the more we CAN do.

For diabetics, getting and staying fit is a high priority. It's essential for managing the disease, and if you're prediabetic, for staving it off. Exercise helps the body respond to insulin, lowers blood sugar levels, improves circulation, burns calories and helps maintain a healthy weight, reduces stress, lessens high blood pressure, controls cholesterol—and the beat goes on. There's almost no end to the benefits of regular physical activity for diabetics.

Or for anyone else, of course. That has been so well established by now that it almost doesn't bear repeating. But it does bear paying attention to.

It doesn't matter what your gig is—the speed bag or the treadmill, the tennis racket or the golf club, hiking up a hill or snowboarding down it, or surfing along the face of a wave—using energy is essential to overall health and is also a way of recharging our lives. There's no other way to do it except to do it. We know that an exercise program should include cardiovascular training, strength training, and stretching. We know we're going to have to sweat. Personally, I love sweating—in a *hamam* in Istanbul or a *shvitz* on the Lower East Side of Manhattan or a sweat lodge in New Mexico or my gym in Brooklyn. It rids the body of waste, and it cools you down. It makes the skin feel great too.

GETTING IT DONE

The only real issue with exercise is getting it done. And the only answer—for people with busy schedules and multiple responsibilities and just not enough hours in the day—is to find the time.

It helps if the exercise is fun, but let's face it: It's not always going to be fun. So take fun out of the equation as a reason for doing exercise—the reason for doing it is that it keeps you alive and safe and healthy—and count fun as a bonus when it happens. There's a real logic to this. I'd rather be surfing off Montauk than running a treadmill in a gym, but running the treadmill makes me a stronger surfer, and that makes the surfing, when I get to it, even better.

For me, I also admit that I am, in this as in just about everything, a competitive dude. Just the way lawyers figure there's maybe a better lawyer out there, or plumbers worry about a better plumber, or chefs like me get our juices going on the idea that there may be better chefs out there, I also get revved when I think about people in better shape. When I see other bodies that are in tip-top condition, and I think how their pancreases are just jamming—and mine isn't!—that's fuel to me. That's when I step up *my* game: I work out harder, I work out more, and then it spreads to other parts of my life and I get that feeling that there is no challenge I can't tackle.

ESPECIALLY FOR DIABETICS

For diabetics, there's another big reason for being almost religiously focused on exercise, although the big reason is just a small number. You know it: your A1C. It is the mother of all blood sugar testing. The one number that, no matter how much you think you may be fooling your doctor or your mother or yourself, won't let you get away with it. This is your reality check, and it smacks you to attention every 90 days. That's how often they tell us we should be tested for A1C— at least four times a year.

Officially, A1C is a hemoglobin that is measured to identify average blood sugar level *over time*. That means it tells you whether or not your blood sugar is within a healthy range. An out-of-balance blood sugar level pretty much foretells heart trouble, kidney trouble, eye trouble, and every other kind of complication to which diabetes makes us vulnerable. That's why monitoring A1C regularly is so important, because there are steps to take to help bring the level back within a healthy range—exercise being a key one of those steps.

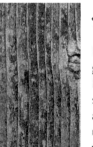

Diabetics and the Sun

I love surfing, paddle boarding, and just general goofing around on the beach, but take note: Diabetics should take special care to avoid sunburn. Research shows that a sunburn actually raises your blood glucose level. So suit up or slather up with a high SPF sunscreen whenever you're out in the sun—in or out of the water.

So every 3 months, we diabetics get checked for our A1C number, aiming and hoping to come in under 7 percent. In fact, the number we're shooting for is around a 6; it is tough work, but it is totally doable. And the closer we are to that little number, the bigger our chances of living the Sweet Life without health complications.

The same goes for blood pressure, the other number that a diabetic has to keep an eye on. If you're diabetic, you know that you need to keep your BP as close to 130 over 80 as possible. Exercise can do it.

So for us, there's really no alternative. We have to jog, ride a bike, swim, run, shoot baskets, do Pilates, whatever—just make sure we do it regularly and without fail. Our health depends on it, and staying alive depends on our health. It's why we're models of healthy living the rest of you would do well to follow. Eat the way diabetics should eat and exercise the way diabetics should exercise, and chances are good you'll live a long, healthy life.

I make exercise my business every day—no days off unless I'm sick. The way my life works is that I am usually at home in New York through the middle of the week, then often on the road. In New York, I know I can get to my gym; on the road, I'm never entirely sure that there will be a gym I can use, or that the gym hours or my own schedule will let me get to it, or that bad weather in Chicago won't paralyze travel and imprison me in an airport for 10 hours. Lots of people who travel on business know what that's about.

For that reason, my idea is to do as much as I can when I can—on the theory that the time may come when I won't get a chance to do it at all. That means on Monday, Tuesday, and Wednesday, I make sure to work out hard and long. A typical hard-and-long workout usually includes a yoga class, close to an hour of cardio work, and some very vigorous muscle-busters focused on upper body and abs. If the schedule for the latter part of the week allows me get to the gym each day, I'll go, but I'll go lighter: maybe an hour total workout, and not as hard: some cardio, stretching, ab work, and push-ups. These are also the kinds of

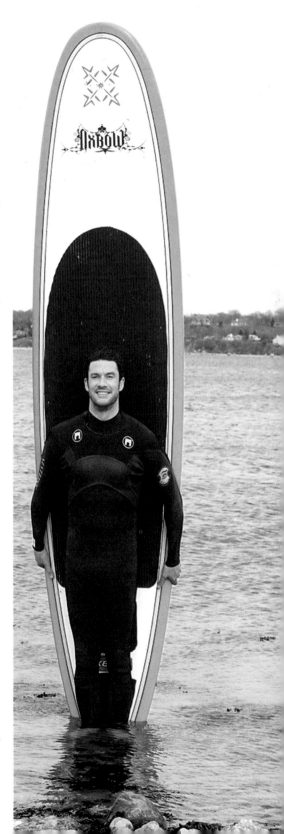

My Exercise Routine

I start every workout with a good 10 minutes of stretching, and I use that time to reflect and focus on the exercise. I call it "getting Zen"—I just try to get all the clutter and cobwebs out of my head and focus on my body and its strength and how the movement feels.

Then I jump on the treadmill for 10 minutes of hard cardio exercise—either running or jogging or walking.

So now my heart rate is up, my lungs are pumping, and I've worked up a bit of a sweat. I'm ready for the yoga that is central to my exercise routine and for the targeted strength training of just about every workout. And when I've finished with that, I always end with another 10 minutes of stretching to unwind and loosen all those muscles.

For me, music is crucial throughout this process, and I recommend it for keeping your mind from wandering back to the office, or over to the spat you had with your significant other, or how angry you are about the news coming out of somewhere or other. Also, it lays down a beat your body will automatically adjust to so you keep on keeping on. I stuff my iPod into a pocket in my sweatpants and just groove, but of course, if what you like is getting down in Downward-Facing Dog, Dr. Dre may not be your cup of tea.

The other thing that's crucial for my exercise routine is to keep changing it up. Otherwise, the second my body realizes that it's on the same old path, it gets lazy and bored—and then I'm just going through useless motions. So while I pretty much stick to the content of the routine, I mix it up—change the order within a workout or over the course of the week.

Here's my typical gym workout schedule; note that each day's workout starts with:

- **A 10-minute clear-the-mind stretch**
- **A 10-minute cardio on the treadmill**

And each ends with:

- **A 10-minute unwinding stretch**

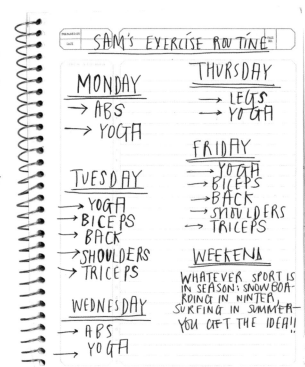

exercises that are easier to do in a hotel gym where the equipment may be limited, or even in the confines of a hotel room.

Wherever and whenever I do it, exercise energizes me. If I can get to it first thing in the morning, I'm amped for the day; the exercise acts like a triple espresso injected directly into the vein. If there's a lull during the day and I can find a way to do a workout, I feel like a phone that's on its last bar and then got plugged in for a recharge: vroom!

And the truth is that my workout is a part of the day I love. The BlackBerry isn't chirping at me or vibrating in my pocket. No one can reach me. Even the city seems to melt away. It's like Sean Astin says in that great speech in *The Goonies*: "Down here, it's our time." When I'm free of everything and focused on keeping my body strong and fit and healthy, that's my time—and it feels great.

STAY FOCUSED, HAVE FUN

One thing I do know is that if exercise is going to count, you have to focus. Making the gym just another place where you multitask misses the point entirely. But it happens. I see people pedaling away on stationary bikes while they text instructions to their assistants back at the office. I see guys on the treadmill, their eyes glued to the stock ticker on the CNBC screen, and they're shouting buy and sell orders to their brokers over their Bluetooth headsets. What's the point? Yeah, their legs are moving, but their stress levels are probably soaring at the same time. The idea is to leave behind all the excess baggage you've picked up during the day—not add to it. Exercise can be mentally rejuvenating as well as physically good for you, but only if you let it.

That means cutting out the distractions and focusing on the sheer physicality of the effort you're expending. In short, sweat the stress out of your body. Pulverize it. Or, if intensity isn't your thing, try endurance. I have a friend who takes a 5-mile walk for exercise. She swears that whatever has been bothering her is out of her system by mile 1 and completely forgotten by mile 2, so what's left is a 3-mile walk for fun and exercise and thinking wonderful thoughts.

REPLENISHING DELICIOUSLY

It's never a good idea to eat right before you exercise, but it's always essential to replenish your body at some point afterward. For diabetics or prediabetics or those hoping never to be either, there's just no getting around the fact that to fuel all that exercise and replenish the body, you need carbs. And carbs, of course, are the things we diabetics have to be particularly careful about. We need to manage the amount of our intake and the kinds of carbs we eat. Even for people for whom diabetes isn't remotely on the radar, a low-carb or at least a managed-carb diet can be useful, especially if they are looking to control their weight. In addition to carbs, having the wherewithal for exercise means you need sufficient protein, lots of fiber, and plenty of water to keep you hydrated. And fatty foods are out.

All those criteria are satisfied by the recipes in this chapter. And so are the taste buds, of course.

You'll get your carbs in the form of low-glycemic-index whole wheat or whole-grain foods like pasta, barley, and spelt, with lots of fruit and veggies. Yum. You'll find protein in tofu and quinoa—one of my favorite foods: a pseudo-grain (it's actually a seed) that is that rare thing, a complete-protein plant food that contains an arsenal of all sorts of other nutrients as well.

Note too that a number of these recipes call for steaming—whether vegetables, grains, or chicken—which avoids the use of fats or oils for sautéing or grilling.

These recipes provide support for those efforts to stay fit and strong and nimble and to achieve and maintain a healthy weight while doing so. For those reasons, these recipes focus on dishes that are low in fat, high in protein and fiber and whole-grain carbohydrates, varied in taste and texture, and of course very, very delicious. These are meals that build muscle and keep you fortified and lean as you play a sport, or work out in the gym, or undertake an outdoor activity—whether it's mowing the lawn or climbing Mount Everest.

And speaking of Mount Everest, a quick word about goji berries, which originally come from the north side of Mount Everest in China. Goji (also grown for centuries in Britain) are dried for consumption and are another superfood, like açai. They are amazingly rich in antioxidants and also provide a taste both tangy and nutty, making goji, in my view, a versatile culinary ingredient, one I use a lot. My Hibiscus and Goji Iced Tea (page 31) makes a soothing energy drink—hot or cold—after a workout or a game of tennis or whatever you do to stay fit. It is my stress-relieving pick-me-up of choice.

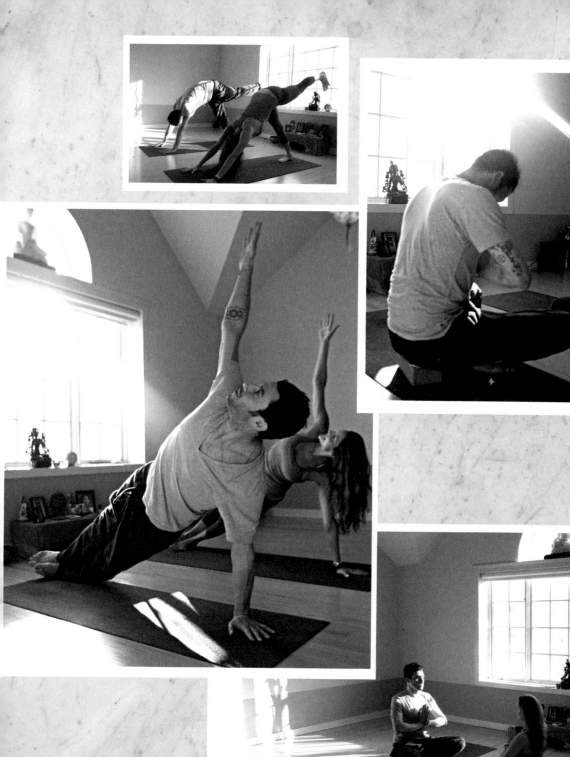

Provençal Salad

 4

This salad is obviously good for you because it's fresh, vibrant, and damn delicious. I love salads like this that are full of big tastes and textures. This has many of the flavors of a classic salade Niçoise and is just as satisfying.

To make the dressing: In a bowl, whisk together the vinegar, lemon juice, agave nectar, Dijon mustard, shallot, garlic, Old Bay seasoning, salt, pepper, and mustard powder. Slowly stream in the oil, whisking constantly. If the consistency is too thick, whisk in 1 tablespoon water.

To make the salad: Place the eggs in a large pot with a tightly fitting lid and fill the pot with cold water, covering the eggs by 1 inch. Cover the pot and bring the water to a boil over medium-high heat. As soon as the water reaches a rolling boil, remove the pot from the heat and let the eggs stand, covered, for 7 minutes. Drain the eggs. When cool enough to handle, shell the eggs under tepid running water and pat dry. Set aside.

Meanwhile, bring a large pot of generously salted water to a simmer over medium-high heat. Add the beans and cook for 30 seconds. With a slotted spoon, transfer the beans to a colander and run them under cold water for 1 minute to stop the cooking and retain their bright green color. Transfer the beans to a large bowl. Keep the cooking water at a simmer.

Add the sweet potatoes to the simmering water and cook until they are fork-tender, 20 to 25 minutes. Drain the potatoes and add to the bowl with the beans.

Add the tomatoes, olives, capers, basil, parsley, radicchio, and arugula and toss to combine well.

Divide the salad among 4 plates and lightly dress with the vinaigrette. Top each serving with 1 egg cut in half so that the yolk runs down the salad.

PER SERVING: 403 calories, 10 g protein, 33 g carbohydrates, 27 g total fat (5 g saturated), 212 mg cholesterol, 5 g fiber, 1,251 mg sodium

DRESSING

- ¼ cup Champagne vinegar
- Juice of 2 lemons
- 1 tablespoon agave nectar
- 1 teaspoon Dijon mustard
- 1 tablespoon diced shallot
- 4 cloves Roasted Garlic (page 93), lightly mashed
- 1 teaspoon Old Bay seasoning
- 1 teaspoon fine sea salt
- 1 teaspoon freshly ground black pepper
- 1 teaspoon mustard powder
- ⅓ cup extra-virgin olive oil

SALAD

- 4 cage-free organic eggs
- ¾ pound green beans, halved
- 2 medium sweet potatoes, peeled and cut into 1-inch cubes
- ½ cup halved cherry tomatoes
- ½ cup kalamata olives, sliced
- 3 tablespoons drained capers
- 2 tablespoons shredded basil
- 2 tablespoons shredded flat-leaf parsley leaves
- 1 large head radicchio, and shredded
- 2 handfuls baby arugula

Spicy Cucumber Salad with Charred Red Onion and Cabbage

 4

Kimchi, a chili-spiced fermented cabbage that is synonymous with Korean food, tastes amazing and is great for you—it's full of healthy bacteria that keep your intestinal tract happy. I sometimes get a bit crazy with it and put it on eggs, hot dogs, or bread, or just eat it on its own as a salad. This isn't a kimchi by any stretch, but it's a variation on the theme—basically just a salad consisting of marinated cucumbers. It's got many refreshing components and some spice to liven things up a bit. It's a great side next to a grilled fish or as part of a potluck spread.

Preheat an outdoor grill or a stovetop grill pan to medium-high heat.

Heat a small skillet over medium-high heat. Add the cumin seeds and toast until fragrant, 15 to 20 seconds. Transfer the toasted seeds to a spice grinder or clean coffee grinder and process until they are finely ground.

In a medium bowl, whisk together the ground cumin, turmeric, 2 tablespoons of the oil, and 1 teaspoon water. Add the onion slices to the bowl, turning to coat well in the marinade. Grill the onions until charred all over, 1 to 2 minutes per side. Set aside.

In a large skillet, heat the remaining 2 tablespoons oil over medium-high heat. Add the ginger, garlic, and cabbage, and cook until the cabbage is wilted, 2 to 3 minutes. Transfer the cabbage mixture to a large bowl and let cool to room temperature.

Add the charred onions, cucumbers, agave nectar, chili paste, and lemon juice. Toss to combine and season to taste with salt and pepper.

PER SERVING: 262 calories, 6 g protein, 30 g carbohydrates, 16 g total fat (2 g saturated), 1 mg cholesterol, 8 g fiber, 86 mg sodium

- 1 teaspoon cumin seeds
- 1 teaspoon turmeric
- 4 tablespoons olive oil
- 1 large red onion, cut crosswise into ½-inch-thick slices
- 1 tablespoon finely chopped fresh ginger
- 2 garlic cloves, smashed and finely chopped
- ½ head napa cabbage, shredded
- 2 large hothouse cucumbers, halved lengthwise and cut crosswise into ¼-inch-thick half-moons
- 2 tablespoons agave nectar
- 1 tablespoon chili paste
- Juice of 2 lemons
- Salt and freshly ground black pepper
- ½ cup hand-torn fresh mint leaves

Stir-Fried Cucumbers with Poppyseeds and Grapefruit

(4-6) For diabetics, grapefruit helps reduce the impact of starches and sweets, so for this and many other reasons, I'm a huge fan. Grapefruits have a lower glycemic load than oranges, so you don't have to use the fruit sparingly; you can get a nice overload of flavor from these gals. They're quite tart, too, so they offer a proper kick-in-the-arse. When you're under the gun timewise and trying to get into health mode, you can definitely use something fast and light like this unusual side dish. Very refreshing, and the warm cucumbers make a flavor twist I really fancy.

In a wok, heat the sesame oil over medium-high heat. Add the onion, garlic, ginger, and cabbage and cook until the onion is translucent and the cabbage has begun to wilt, 3 to 4 minutes.

Toss in the cucumbers and poppyseeds and cook, stirring constantly, for 1 minute. Add the soy sauce and stir-fry for 1 minute. Transfer the vegetables to a serving bowl or plate and sprinkle with the grapefruit zest and juice. Season to taste with salt and pepper.

PER SERVING: 165 calories, 4 g protein, 15 g carbohydrates, 12 g total fat (2 g saturated), 0 mg cholesterol, 4 g fiber, 272 mg sodium

- 3 tablespoons toasted sesame oil
- 1 Vidalia or yellow onion, thinly sliced
- 4 garlic cloves, smashed and finely chopped
- 2 tablespoons finely chopped fresh ginger
- 1 cup finely shredded green cabbage
- 2 hothouse cucumbers, cut crosswise into ¼-inch-thick half-moons
- 1 tablespoon poppyseeds
- 2 tablespoons reduced-sodium soy sauce
- 1 teaspoon grated zest and the juice of 1 Ruby Red grapefruit (or 2 pomelos, if in season)
- Salt and freshly ground black pepper

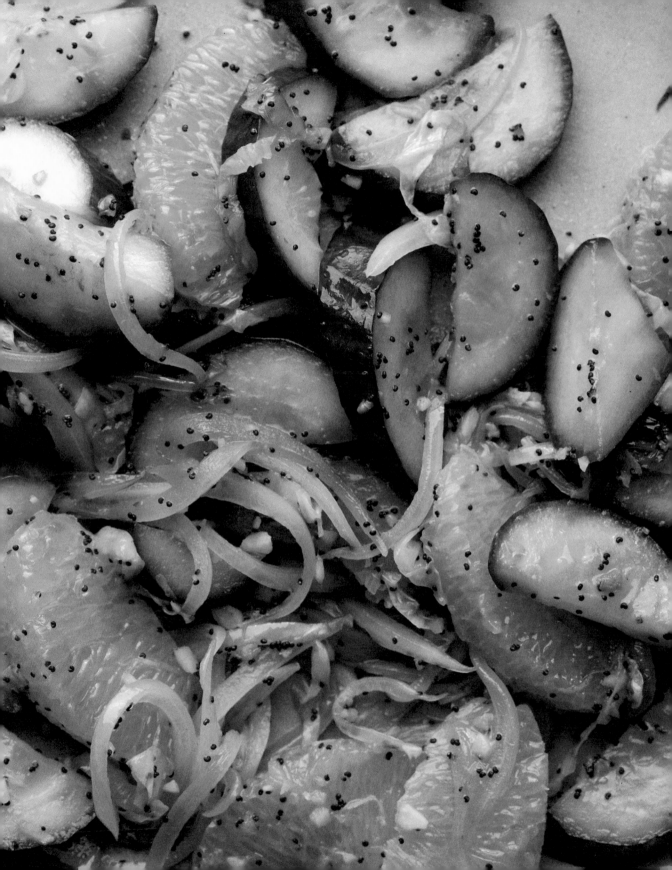

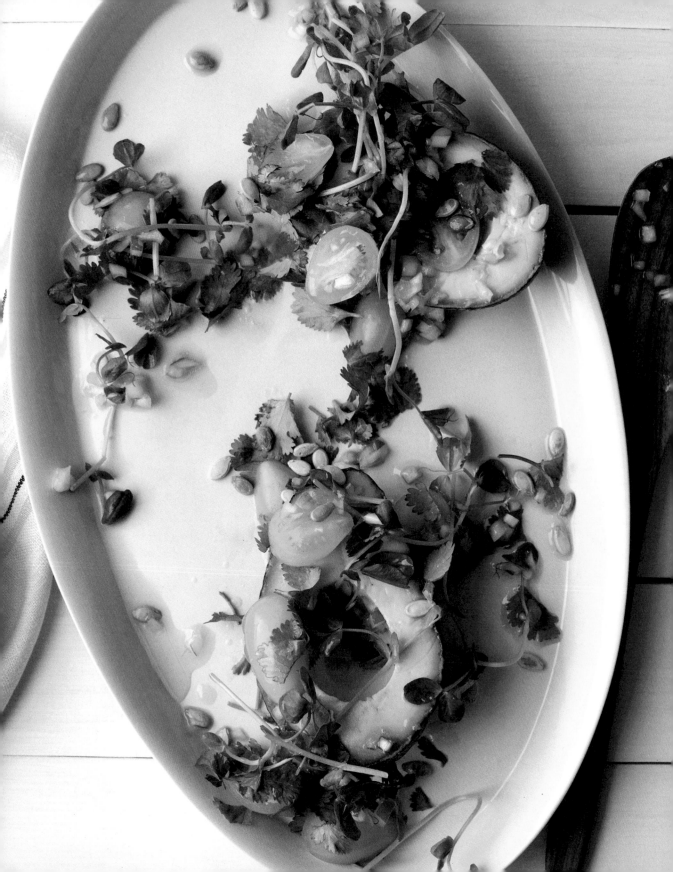

Avocado with Roasted Watermelon Seeds and Pea Shoot Salad

This is a chick dish for sure. Women seem to love avocados—whether it's guacamole and chips and fruity avocado salads, or in masks and eye creams and oils for their skin. Hey, so do I. Avocado is refreshing, and it has a definite cooling effect. But beyond all those attractive features, avocados are nutritional heavyweights. The American Heart Association recommends that 30 percent of your daily calories should come from fat, primarily unsaturated fat. Avocado's got it. The AHA also recommends 5 servings of fruits and veggies daily, and avocado certainly counts as a fruit. And watermelon seeds—most often overlooked but high in protein and B vitamins—are delicious when roasted and seasoned well. I make this dish for you, ladies—and for men who like avocadoes as much as I do. C'mon, I know you're out there.

If using fresh (untoasted) watermelon seeds or plain hulled pumpkin or sunflower seeds, start by roasting the seeds. Heat 2 tablespoons of the oil in a medium skillet over medium heat. Add the seeds and cook until you can smell their nutty aroma, 2 to 3 minutes. Set aside to cool.

In a large bowl, combine the pea shoots, cilantro, tomatoes, and onion. In a small bowl, whisk together the lemon zest and juice, vinegar, garlic, and remaining 4 tablespoons oil. Add the vinaigrette to the pea shoot mixture and toss well to combine.

Halve the avocados, pit, and peel. Place 1 avocado half on each of 4 plates and top each serving with some of the pea shoot salad. Season to taste with salt and pepper.

PER SERVING: 410 calories, 7 g protein, 22 g carbohydrates, 36 g total fat (5 g saturated), 0 mg cholesterol, 10 g fiber, 52 mg sodium

⅓ cup raw or roasted watermelon seeds, pumpkin seeds (pepitas), or sunflower seeds

6 tablespoons olive oil

1 pound pea shoots

1 cup tightly packed hand-torn fresh cilantro

1 pint pear tomatoes or cherry tomatoes, halved

1 large red onion, finely diced

Grated zest and juice of 4 lemons

3 tablespoons red wine vinegar

1 garlic clove, smashed and finely chopped

2 Hass avocados

Salt and freshly ground black pepper

Carrot Salad with Tahini and Orange

Because people with diabetes are concerned with the glycemic load (GL) of foods, or the amount of sugar per serving, it's good to know that this carrot salad has a very low GL *and* a lot of flavor. The tahini, which is ground sesame seeds, adds a dense nuttiness similar to that of peanut butter. Even for a salad, it's hearty—great with a lager on a fall afternoon.

Bring a large pot of water to a boil and fill a large bowl with ice water. Add the carrots to the boiling water and cook until they are crisp-tender, 1 to 2 minutes; they should still be crunchy. Drain and transfer the carrots to the bowl of ice water to cool and stop the cooking. Drain the carrots well and set them aside.

In a large skillet, heat the garlic oil over medium-high heat. Add the onion, garlic, and ginger and cook, stirring frequently, until the onions are translucent, 2 to 3 minutes. Add 3 tablespoons water, the vinegar, tahini, agave nectar, and harissa. Toss the ingredients well. Transfer the vinaigrette to a serving bowl.

Add the carrots to the bowl and mix well. Sprinkle with 1 tablespoon of the orange zest, the orange juice, and the cilantro. Toss again and serve.

PER SERVING: 187 calories, 2 g protein, 19 g carbohydrates, 13 g total fat (2 g saturated), 0 mg cholesterol, 3 g fiber, 66 mg sodium

6 carrots, cut into ½-inch pieces

3 tablespoons Roasted Garlic Oil (page 93)

½ red onion, diced

3 garlic cloves, smashed and finely chopped

2 tablespoons finely chopped fresh ginger

1 tablespoon white wine vinegar

1 tablespoon tahini

1 tablespoon agave nectar

1 teaspoon harissa

Grated zest and juice of 1 orange

2 tablespoons chopped fresh cilantro

Couscous with Fennel, Coconut, and Pine Nuts

Coconuts are the answer to everything, aren't they? From one funky looking, brown, hairy package you get meat, juice, milk, and oil that are not only good eating, they're used to treat colds, skin infections, even stomachaches. The best part, though—obviously—is the taste and aroma of coconut in a dish like this one. I've always called coconut The Enabler, because it allows the other ingredients in the recipe to stand out as well. This is an outstanding meatless entrée just as is, but it can also double as a side dish for a grilled meat or fish entrée. If Italian pine nuts are too pricey, look for Chinese pine nuts, which are significantly less expensive.

In a medium saucepan, bring the almond milk and broth to a simmer over medium heat on a back burner.

Meanwhile, on a front burner, heat the oil in another medium saucepan over medium-high heat. Add the fennel, onion, garlic, pine nuts, and coconut. Cook about 2 minutes, then add the couscous and cook, stirring vigorously, until toasted and golden brown. Remove from the heat and transfer the couscous mixture to a large bowl.

Pour the hot almond milk-broth mixture over the couscous in the bowl. Stir in the scallions and fluff the couscous with a fork. Cover the bowl tightly with plastic wrap and let the couscous steam until all of the liquid is absorbed, about 20 minutes.

Remove the plastic wrap and sprinkle the couscous with the lemon juice. If the couscous turns out too al dente for your taste, return it to the saucepan, add ½ cup water, and cook on medium-high heat until it reaches the desired texture.

1 cup almond milk

½ cup low-sodium chicken broth

3 tablespoons olive oil

1 large fennel bulb (about 1 pound), stalks discarded, cored, and thinly sliced

1 yellow or Vidalia onion, diced

4 garlic cloves, smashed and chopped

½ cup pine nuts

¼ cup unsweetened shredded coconut

1 cup Israeli couscous

2 scallions, thinly sliced

Juice of 2 lemons

PER SERVING: 459 calories, 11 g protein, 38 g carbohydrates, 16 g total fat (2 g saturated), 0 mg cholesterol, 5 g fiber, 174 mg sodium

Chickpea Tabbouleh with Fuji Apple

Eating tabbouleh is a great way to get your antioxidants! Pound for pound, parsley, the main ingredient in tabbouleh, contains three times as much vitamin C as oranges, has twice as much iron as spinach, and is also an excellent source of folate, vitamin K, and vitamin A. And you know what they say about an apple a day . . .

Stir together the bulgur and salt in a large heatproof bowl. Pour the boiling water over the bulgur, stir, cover the bowl with plastic wrap, and let stand until the water has been absorbed and the bulgur is tender, about 20 minutes.

Add the parsley, mint, chickpeas, scallions, tomatoes, oil, and lemon zest and juice, and toss to mix. Season lightly with salt and pepper and toss again. Let the tabbouleh stand for about 10 minutes, or until it has cooled to room temperature. Just before serving, stir in the apples.

PER SERVING: 266 calories, 7 g protein, 38 g carbohydrates, 12 g total fat (2 g saturated), 0 mg cholesterol, 9 g fiber, 374 mg sodium

½ cup bulgur

½ teaspoon fine sea salt

1 cup boiling water

1 cup loosely packed chopped flat-leaf parsley

1 cup loosely packed chopped fresh mint leaves

1 can (15 ounces) chickpeas, rinsed and drained

2 scallions, thinly sliced

4 medium vine-ripened tomatoes, seeded and chopped

3 tablespoons olive oil

Grated zest and juice of 2 lemons

Freshly ground black pepper

1 Fuji apple, diced (cut just before serving so it doesn't oxidize)

Spelt with Pea Shoots, Parsley, and Pickled Oranges

 6–8

Spelt is the nuttiest of grains, filled with protein and B vitamins. You can use this as a side dish or sub in spelt wherever you'd like something other than rice or potato. I love all the green in this recipe; it makes it taste so fresh and clean, which means you feel fresh and clean from eating it. The quick pickling I use on the oranges you can use on many things; try it with apple or pears or even cherry tomatoes!

To pickle the oranges: Using a sharp knife, slice off all the peel and white pith from both oranges. Cut down along the membranes toward the center of the orange to release the individual segments. Place the orange segments in a large airtight container. Add ⅓ cup cold water, the sweetener, cinnamon stick, pepper flakes, and vinegar, and swirl gently to combine. Cover the container and refrigerate for at least 2 hours or overnight.

To cook the spelt: In a large pot, bring the broth and ½ cup water to a boil over medium-high heat. Add the spelt, reduce to a simmer, cover, and cook until the berries are tender, 25 to 30 minutes. Drain and transfer the cooked spelt to a large bowl.

In a large skillet, heat the garlic oil over medium-high heat. Add the onion, fresh fennel, ginger, and fennel seeds and cook until the onion is translucent and the fennel has softened, 2 to 3 minutes. Set aside to cool to room temperature, about 20 minutes.

Add the cooled onion mixture to the spelt, along with the pea shoots, parsley, mint, olive oil, tamari, and vinegar. Fluff the mixture with a fork to combine. Season to taste with salt and pepper.

When ready to serve, remove the pickled oranges from the refrigerator. Transfer the spelt mixture to a serving platter or individual dishes and top with the pickled orange segments and a few spoonfuls of the pickling liquid.

PER SERVING: 261 calories, 7 g protein, 33 g carbohydrates, 13 g total fat (2 g saturated), 0 mg cholesterol, 6 g fiber, 547 mg sodium

PICKLED ORANGES

- 2 **navel oranges**
- 1 **tablespoon granulated stevia extract, or to taste**
- 1 **cinnamon stick**
- 1 **teaspoon red pepper flakes**
- 3 **tablespoons white wine vinegar**

SPELT AND PEA SHOOTS

- 2 **cups low-sodium chicken broth**
- 1 **cup spelt berries**
- 2 **tablespoons Roasted Garlic Oil (page 93)**
- ¼ **cup diced red onion**
- 1 **small fennel bulb, trimmed, cored, and finely chopped**
- 1 **tablespoon grated ginger**
- 1 **tablespoon fennel seeds**
- 1 **cup pea shoots**
- ½ **cup flat-leaf parsley leaves**
- ¼ **cup fresh mint leaves**
- 3 **tablespoons extra-virgin olive oil**
- 2 **tablespoons tamari**
- 1 **tablespoon red wine vinegar**
  Salt and freshly ground black pepper

Quinoa with Tofu, Lemongrass, and Lime

 4

Quinoa is a complete protein. That means it is totally badass. Complete proteins are so rare in plant foods: Quinoa contains all of the necessary amino acids for feeling and looking great. A lot of people assume that quinoa is "just" a side dish, to be treated sort of like a rice accompaniment. But for me, its texture, its ability to receive seasonings and interact with other ingredients, and its formidable nutritional value all mean that it ranks high on the list. I like to feature it at the taste center of many meals. I eat quinoa at least three times a week. You should, too; it's so damn good for you.

In a medium saucepan, heat 2 tablespoons of the oil over medium heat. Add the shallot, garlic, lemongrass, ginger, coriander seeds, and cumin and cook, stirring frequently, until the shallot is translucent and the garlic and ginger have softened, 2 to 3 minutes.

Add the broth, lime zest and juice, and quinoa. Bring to a boil, cover the pan, and simmer for 12 minutes. Uncover, give it one good stir, then re-cover and cook until the liquid is absorbed and the quinoa is tender, about 3 minutes. Remove from the heat and season to taste with salt and pepper.

Meanwhile, in a medium skillet, heat the remaining 1 tablespoon oil over medium heat. Place the slices of tofu in the hot oil and cook, turning, until golden brown, 3 to 4 minutes per side.

Divide the quinoa among 4 shallow bowls, top each serving with a slice of tofu, and garnish with the cilantro.

PER SERVING: 347 calories, 15 g protein, 38 g carbohydrates, 16 g total fat (2 g saturated), 0 mg cholesterol, 5 g fiber, 286 mg sodium

- 3 tablespoons olive oil
- 1 shallot, finely diced
- 4 garlic cloves, smashed and finely chopped
- 3 tablespoons finely chopped fresh lemongrass
- 2 tablespoons finely chopped fresh ginger
- 1 tablespoon coriander seeds
- 1 teaspoon ground cumin
- 2 cups low-sodium chicken broth

  Grated zest and juice of 2 limes
- 1 cup quinoa, rinsed

  Salt and freshly ground black pepper
- 8 ounces extra-firm tofu, cut into 4 slices
- ½ cup loosely packed hand-torn fresh cilantro

Spaghetti Squash with Marinara, Parmesan, and Basil

There's no getting around the fact that pasta, whether whole wheat, gluten-free, or whatever, is high in carbs—about 42 grams per serving. Once in awhile, especially on an active day, that's okay; the rest of the time, you'll get great pasta flavors from this dish without the carbs. Play with this dish. Think about other components you can add or about what to subtract to fit your personal needs or tastes a bit more. Maybe you have a big family and you want a protein in there. Okay, so roast a whole chicken or fish and top the dish with the pulled meat. It's a blank canvas—have at it.

To make the marinara: In a medium saucepan, heat the oil over medium-high heat. Add the onion, garlic, and carrots and cook until the vegetables are soft and lightly browned, 2 to 3 minutes. Drain off half of the juice from the canned tomatoes and discard. Add the tomatoes and remaining juice to the pan and bring the sauce to a boil. Reduce to a simmer and cook for at least 30 minutes or up to 2 hours if you have the time and want a deeper more concentrated flavor. Just before using, stir in the basil and thyme and season to taste with salt and pepper.

To cook the squash: Preheat the oven to 400°F. Halve the squash lengthwise, drizzle with 1/2 tablespoon of the oil, and place cut side down in a roasting pan. Roast for 50 minutes or until tender when pierced with a fork. Cool for 20 minutes, then discard the seeds. Use a fork to scrape the strands of squash into a mixing bowl. Add the olives, remaining oil, pepper flakes, salt, and black pepper and stir to combine.

Spread the marinara in the bottom of a serving dish, spoon the squash on top, and sprinkle with the sliced basil and Parmesan.

PER SERVING: 266 calories, 10 g protein, 33 g carbohydrates, 14 g total fat (3 g saturated), 4 mg cholesterol, 7 g fiber, 806 mg sodium

MARINARA

- 2 tablespoons olive oil
- 1 small yellow onion, chopped
- 4 garlic cloves, finely chopped
- 2 carrots, finely chopped
- 1 can (28 ounces) crushed San Marzano tomatoes
- ¼ cup hand-torn fresh basil
- 2 tablespoons fresh thyme leaves
- Salt and freshly ground black pepper

SQUASH

- 1 medium spaghetti squash
- 1½ tablespoons olive oil
- ¼ cup chopped kalamata olives
- ½ teaspoon red pepper flakes
- ½ teaspoon fine sea salt
- ¼ teaspoon freshly ground black pepper
- ½ cup thinly sliced fresh basil
- ¼ cup grated Parmesan cheese

whole wheat Spaghetti with Fennel, Strawberries, and Pancetta

 6

This dish is strange, I admit, but *it totally works.* You get great texture from the crunch of the toasted pasta, savory notes from the fennel, and nice porky aftertones that all make it worth the weirdness. Something else that makes it worthwhile: strawberries. The most marketable and popular berry in the world, they are also a huge source of phenols, heart-protective antioxidants. That's a mouthful. And while I know that pancetta has a higher fat content than other proteins, when you taste this, you may just forgive yourself . . . Besides, you don't need to add pancetta every time; sub in another vegetable or protein to put your own spin on the dish. That's playing with your food, and I appreciate that.

Heat the oil in a large skillet over medium-high heat. Break the pasta strands in thirds, add to the skillet, and toast until golden brown, about 2½ minutes; don't let the pasta burn. Bring a large pot of heavily salted water to a boil over high heat. Add the spaghetti and cook until just al dente, 6 to 8 minutes. Drain the spaghetti in a colander, run it under cold water to cool and stop the cooking, and transfer the pasta to a large serving bowl. Add the strawberries, basil, rosemary, and olive oil and toss to coat.

In a medium skillet, heat the garlic oil over medium-high heat. Add the pancetta and cook until golden brown, about 4 minutes. Add the roasted garlic, shallots, fennel, and pepper flakes and cook until the shallots are translucent and the fennel begins to soften, 2 to 3 minutes. Add the wine and cook for 2 minutes, scraping up the browned bits from the bottom to deglaze the pan. Add the broth and cook for 2 minutes to heat through.

Pour the sauce from the pan over the pasta, tossing and combining well. Squeeze the lemon juice over the top.

PER SERVING: 437 calories, 15 g protein, 65 g carbohydrates, 17 g total fat (4 g saturated), 0 mg cholesterol, 12 g fiber, 643 mg sodium

- **2 tablespoons olive oil**
- **12 ounces whole wheat spaghetti**
- **1 cup quartered strawberries**
- **¾ cup loosely packed hand-torn fresh basil**
- **2 tablespoons chopped fresh rosemary**
- **1 tablespoon extra-virgin olive oil**
- **1 tablespoon Roasted Garlic Oil (page 93)**
- **¼ pound pancetta, diced**
- **8 cloves Roasted Garlic (page 93), lightly mashed**
- **2 shallots, diced**
- **1 large fennel bulb (about 1 pound), stalks discarded, cored, and cut into slivers**
- **1 teaspoon red pepper flakes**
- **1 cup dry white wine**
- **¼ cup low-sodium chicken broth**
- **2 lemons, halved**

Linguine with whole clams

Most linguines with clam sauce have far too much linguine and not enough clams for this mollusk lover; by upping the clams and cutting the pasta to a reasonable 2 ounces per person I've not only made it more diabetic-friendly, I've let the seafood take center stage. If you want to skip the carbs altogether, or if you want a change of pace one evening, there's a light alternative to this recipe: Omit the pasta and add some cubed squash or ribbons of zucchini instead.

Bring a medium pot of water to a boil. Add the pasta and cook according to the package directions. Drain the pasta, transfer it to a large serving bowl, and toss it with the parsley and extra-virgin olive oil to prevent it from sticking together. Set the pasta aside.

In a large skillet, heat the regular olive oil over medium-high heat. Add the garlic, celery, shallot, and fennel seeds and cook, stirring constantly, until the garlic and celery are translucent, 2 to 3 minutes. Add the clam juice, wine, and Old Bay and stir to combine. Add the clams, cover the pan, and cook until the clams open, 4 to 6 minutes. Discard any unopened shells.

Pour the clams and broth over the linguine. Sprinkle with the lemon juice and toss the pasta with tongs to mix it all together. Serve hot.

PER SERVING: 374 calories, 21 g protein, 55 g carbohydrates, 10 g total fat (2 g saturated), 29 mg cholesterol, 8 g fiber, 740 mg sodium

½ **pound whole wheat linguine**

½ **cup loosely packed hand-torn flat-leaf parsley**

1 **teaspoon extra-virgin olive oil**

2 **tablespoons olive oil**

6 **garlic cloves, smashed and finely chopped**

4 **celery ribs, finely chopped**

1 **shallot, finely chopped**

1 **tablespoon fennel seeds**

1 **cup bottled clam juice**

2 **tablespoons dry white wine**

1 **tablespoon Old Bay seasoning**

3 **dozen Manila or Little Neck clams, scrubbed**

Juice of 2 lemons

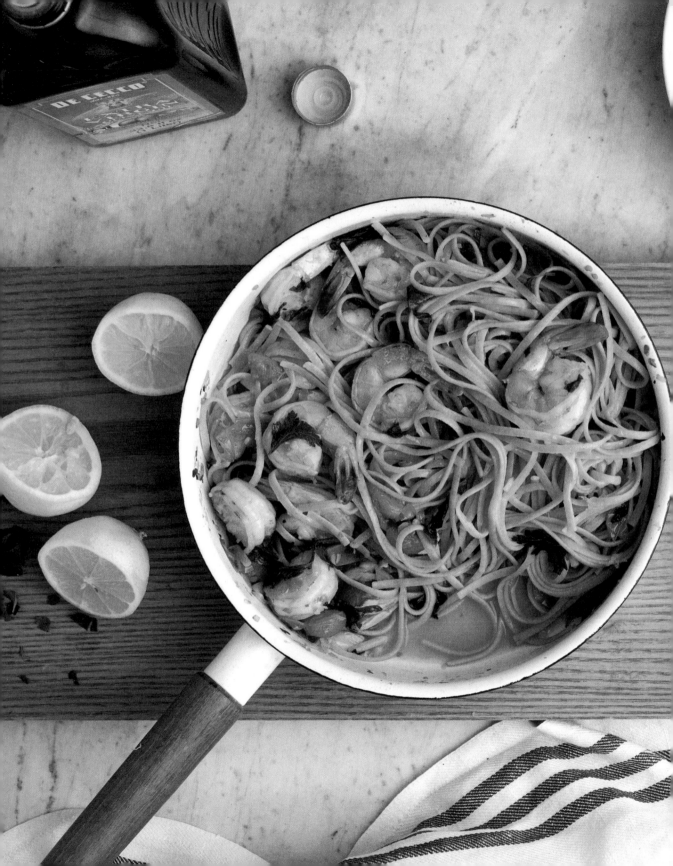

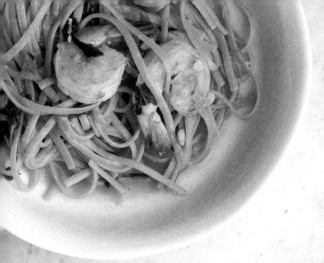

Pan-Roasted Shrimp with Whole Wheat Linguine

6 The great thing about a dish like linguine with some kind of seafood "sauce" is that you can play with it endlessly. This dish is soooo simple, so healthy, so delicious. And it takes almost no time at all to prepare and cook.

Bring a large pot of water to a boil. Add the linguine and cook according to the package directions. Drain well.

Meanwhile, in a large skillet, heat the oil over medium-high heat. Add the garlic, shallots, and pepper flakes and cook until aromatic, 1 to 2 minutes. Add the shrimp and cook until the shrimp start to turn pink, about 1½ minutes. Add the wine and bring to a boil. Reduce the heat to medium-low and cook until the liquid is reduced by half, 2 to 3 minutes. Add the cherry tomatoes and broth to the pan and bring to a simmer.

Add the pasta to the pan, tossing with tongs to coat well with the liquid, then add the parsley and basil and toss once more. Season to taste with salt and pepper, and sprinkle with the lemon zest and juice.

PER SERVING: 400 calories, 33 g protein, 53 g carbohydrates, 8 g total fat (1 g saturated), 172 mg cholesterol, 8 g fiber, 344 mg sodium

- **12** ounces whole wheat linguine
- **2** tablespoons olive oil
- **6** garlic cloves, smashed and finely chopped
- **2** shallots, diced
- **1½** teaspoons red pepper flakes
- **1½** pounds large shrimp, peeled and deveined
- **⅓** cup dry white wine
- **1** cup cherry tomatoes or grape tomatoes
- **1** cup low-sodium chicken broth
- **¼** cup hand-torn flat-leaf parsley leaves
- **¼** cup hand-torn fresh basil leaves

  Salt and freshly ground black pepper

  Grated zest and juice of 1 lemon

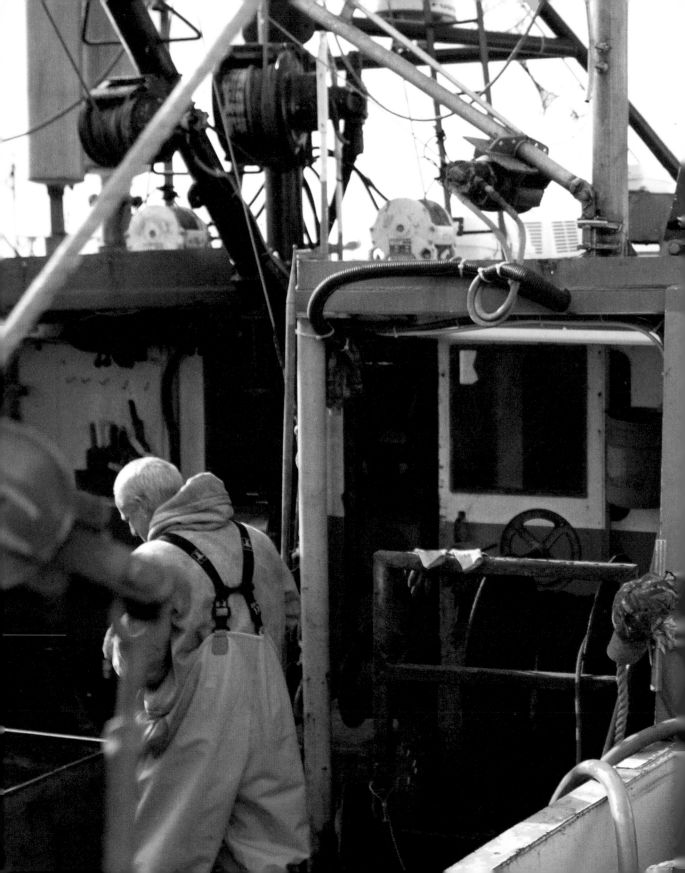

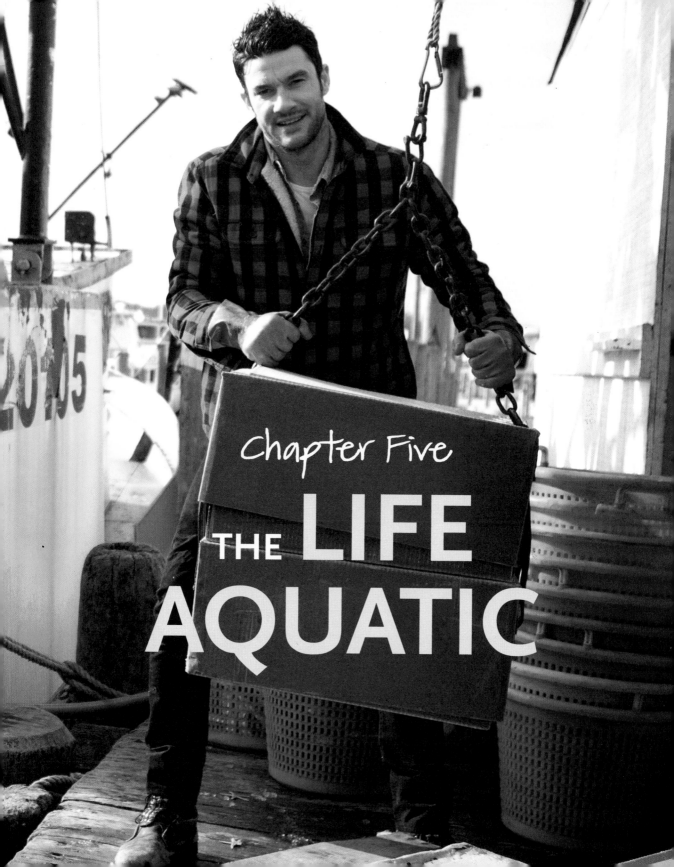

Chapter Five

THE LIFE
AQUATIC

RECIPES
easy fish and seafood

'm a water baby, happiest and at my best on the beach or on the bank of a river or stream. I grew up on the Carolina coast, a coastline dotted with islands and drained by bays and swamps and rivers, and I learned to fish before I learned to read. I remember fishing with my pal Matty, the two of us trying to reel in shark and snapper and bass on our kid-sized reels or going after blue crab on a line or shrimp with an improvised net. The shrimp were tiny, and we used them mostly for bait. But sometimes we'd get hungry enough to grab a handful of them, crack the heads, and eat them right out of the water. Small and crunchy and super-salty, they were like a South Carolina version of potato chips—the perfect snack. And one of the first meals I ever "created" from scratch.

Now I live in one of the world's greatest ports, and I'm the executive chef at two fish and seafood restaurants, so I spend a good part of my waking hours thinking about how to make a good thing better. Freshwater fish, saltwater fish, big fish, little fish, shellfish or scales: If it lives in water, it is my favorite food to eat and my favorite food to cook, and that's what the recipes in this chapter are all about.

Perhaps the best part about eating fish is that it is so very good for us. Rich in vitamins, minerals, and omega-3 fatty acids, fish is above all a vital source of protein—essential for life—for all the world's population. For diabetics, however, it is probably our best source of protein because it tends to be lower in calories than many other sources of protein while acting *against* insulin resistance and *for* heart health. The omega-3 fatty acids in fish, in particular, seem to help lower blood pressure and triglyceride

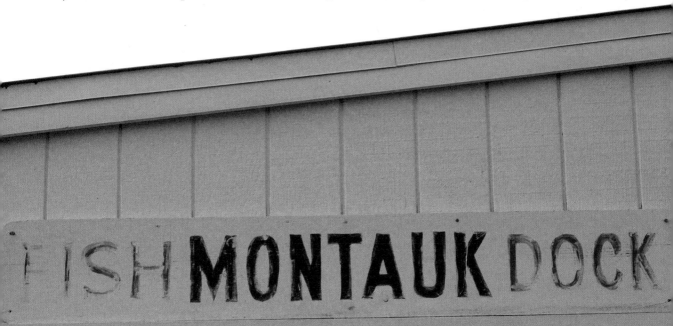

concentrations and to combat potential circulation problems. Fish even helps protect against kidney disease, something it doesn't do for nondiabetics. It's nice to be one up for something, isn't it?

These essential health benefits—not just those for diabetics but all the benefits for everyone—have been available and readily accessible to anyone living near a body of water since the beginning of time. And fish has long been and remains a critical source of protein in places where other sources of animal protein—like cattle—are scarce. Knowing this, shouldn't we be taking very, very good care of our oceans and waterways and of the creatures that inhabit them?

Sadly, we're not. And the consequences of that failure are something I'm passionate about—as a fish-lover and a chef, as a water sportsman, and as someone who loves oceans and rivers and streams and believes we need to pay more attention to what we're doing to our planet. It's why I'm so committed to the concept of sustainable seafood, a concept I try to advance every day in my work as a chef, a concept embodied by all the recipes in this chapter.

SUSTAINABLE SEAFOOD

We used to think the sea's bounty was limitless, but population growth and industrialized fishing are depleting fish stocks everywhere. Some industrialized tuna fishing enterprises, for example, using huge netting techniques, wastefully sweep up and kill all sorts of other fish—swordfish and dolphin, for example—in their by-catch just to get enough albacore to put into cans. It's the collateral damage of the fishing industry, and it has a frightening long-term impact for these fish populations, more and more of which are simply vanishing from the sea. Meanwhile, aquaculture—fish farming—has potential problems, too; we have to be very careful that it doesn't further risk the health of already threatened wild fish populations.

This is why sustainability is the ruling principle of the way I work and why I have made sustainable seafood my "brand." And because so many more people care about sustainability these days, my obsessiveness over sourcing, preparing, cooking, and serving fish looks a lot less like craziness and a lot more like an essential professional tool. Customers at Imperial No. 9 and The Surf Lodge know they are coming to an eco-responsible restaurant; they know that sense of responsibility means food that not only tastes good, but that does no harm to other species or to the planet. Granted, you won't be cooking for a paying public, but you're actually cooking for an even more important group of "guests"— yourself and your family. You want to be sure you're giving them the highest-quality, healthiest food there is. Where fish and seafood are concerned, that means "sustainable." And you can ensure sustainability by following the same principles we use in our restaurants, adapting them to your own practices.

RESEARCH AND MORE RESEARCH

For anyone who may think that being a chef is just about what happens in the kitchen, let me assure you that it isn't. It starts with research, and for professionals in the business, the research never lets up. At the restaurant we keep on top of national and local issues on a regular basis through websites like the Clean Ocean Action, which focuses on improving the quality of the waters of the New York and New Jersey coasts, and our mainstay, Seafood Watch (see page 131). We're also hooked into—no pun intended—the fish advisories of the federal Environmental Protection Agency and the food safety alerts and environmental assessments regularly issued by the Food and Drug Administration.

I am on my computer and checking my BlackBerry almost around the clock getting the latest alerts about a species that's just been declared endangered or about the most recent pollution spill or the like. All of this is an ongoing and essential task, and it is bound to remain one until the seas and streams of our planet get permanently clean—which is not going to be anytime soon.

Choosing species of fish and seafood we know are safe to eat is just the first step; next is making sure that we're getting the highest quality fish and seafood for the restaurants. For that, I follow two operating principles that you should observe as well: traceability and accountability. This means knowing as much as you can about where and how the fish was caught and that the people purveying the fish are accountable for how it was caught.

I actually know the fishermen who provide fish to my restaurant. I've met the guys who are out there in the boat bringing in the crabs. I've talked to the people catching the bass or haddock, and I've assured myself that they do it with rod and line. Why would you not want to know who caught the fish you're eating and how and where it was caught?

In addition, we train the entire staff to be knowledgeable and comfortable speaking about what fish and shellfish we offer and what species we do not offer—and why. We regularly offer courses on sustainable seafood to make sure our waiters and cooks know how to talk about these issues with diners. We want them to understand that we have a responsibility to ensure that there be seafood for future generations, that we support environmentally responsible fishing and aquaculture, that we try to promote interest in ocean-friendly sea-food, and that we want to give imperiled species a break so they can recover and thrive once again—all of which may mean we won't be able to serve a particular species, no matter how popular it is.

So at The Surf Lodge, we'll stick to local oysters from Montauk caught by my friend Mike and local Montauk clams from my friend Damon. For Imperial No. 9, there's a fisherman I can reach by cell phone who will bring me only line-caught "green light" fish off the coast of Block Island. These are fish at the lower end of the food chain, and by going after them we're leaving plenty of other species for the large predator fish to find and eat—a key goal because these magnificent creatures are now vanishing rapidly from our oceans.

We also have been in contact with some of the premier fish farms in the world as well. I used to be against using farm-raised fish until I looked deeper into the eco-friendly methods and feeds the best of these farms use. And I've found many of them can provide me with ingredients that are both sustainably produced and have great flavor.

For example, I've found Peruvian lantern scallops cultivated in clean Pacific waters on a low-impact, innovative farm using the traditional off-bottom, Japanese lantern method. The operation is powered with clean alternative fuels and has zero impact on the sea floor. This is a cutting-edge, environmentally responsible scallop farm, and the scallops are delicious.

EATING AND COOKING FISH

Once you've got a good, very fresh piece of fish, or pile of shellfish, the point is to keep it clean and keep it simple. I learned this style of cooking, as most people do, at home—my mother is an exceptional cook. Clam chowders, spaghetti and clams, insanely good fresh tuna melts on rye: The ingredients were always fresh and clean, the cooking simple and delicious. My mom's clam chowder was the best—still is, flavored with fresh local plum clams, bacon, and celery seed. My chowder (see page 78) is the same idea, just tweaked with a modern touch: almond milk! It's got phenomenal health benefits and also works wonders to give the chowder a rich nutty balance while not trumping the clam flavor—just elevating it a touch. It's a modern tweak that make sense to me and, I hope, will to you as well.

The striped bass in this chapter is a perfect case in point. In the summer, when the tomatoes were ripe on the vine, my mom would broil some sort of fresh fish and serve it simply over sliced fresh Carolina tomatoes. My stepfather, Joey, and I loved it. So when The Surf Lodge was born, it seemed natural to pair the abundant striped bass that run off Montauk in the summer months with the delicious tomatoes that grow in nearby Amagansett. At Surf Lodge we cook it *a la plancha*—seared on a very hot metal grill—

Seafood Watch

At both my restaurants, we're addicted to the Seafood Watch of the Monterey Bay Aquarium. Located in Monterey, California—and one of the great aquariums to visit—it keeps tabs on overfishing, illegal and unregulated fishing, pollution and other forms of habitat damage, accidental catches of species, and more, and it sends out regular color-coded bulletins. Red-alert species are fish to avoid, orange is for good alternatives, and green is for best choices: sustainable seafood that is clean and not overfished or depleting other stocks.

And here's the great news: The Seafood Watch is online, available to all at http://www.montereybayaquarium. org/cr/seafoodwatch.aspx. The site even lets you download a mobile app for your smartphone. This means that whether you're shopping in the market for fish or browsing the seafood menu at a restaurant, you have access to the latest data on the fish that are good for both you and the oceans; just click it on your phone. Both of the restaurants I'm involved with follow the guidelines of that program, pledging as much as possible to serve nothing that appears on the Aquarium's Seafood Watch "Avoid" list and I challenge you to make the same pledge for the food you cook and serve at home. It just makes good sense on every level.

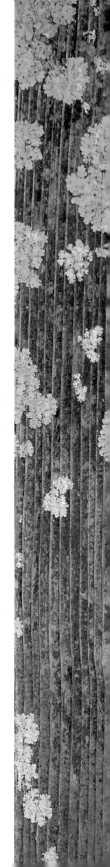

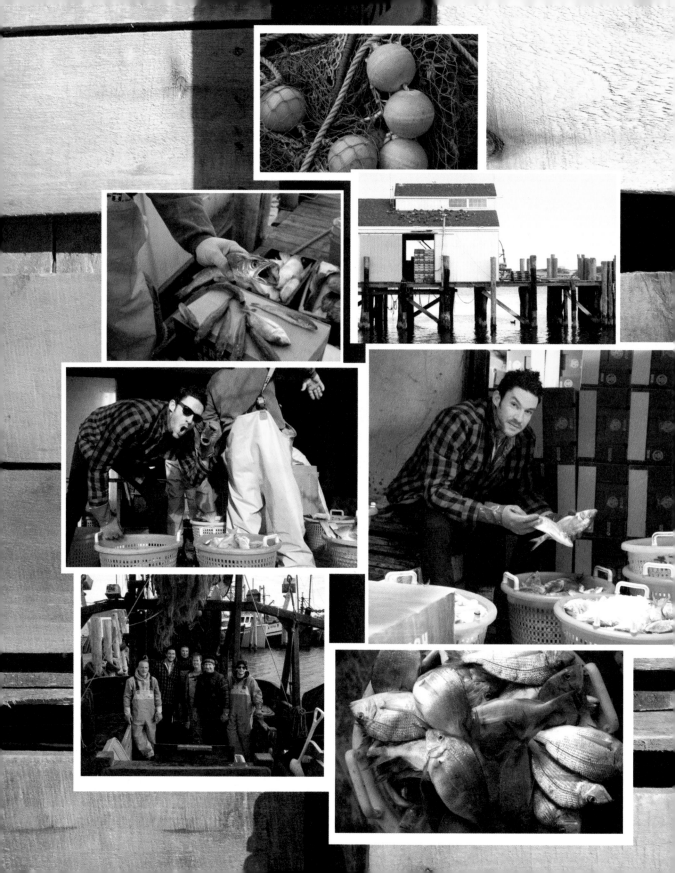

then, instead of serving the tomatoes raw, we sauté them just to open up the natural sweetness a bit, and we work in some toasted garlic to start a full-blown summer love affair. There's a truth that can't be too often repeated, and it's that cooking and eating a fish that was caught just hours before it reaches your plate can be life changing. It changed and molded my life and helped make me the chef I am today. (For that, I thank Matty and his Mama Jimi for all those summers of "instruction" destroying his mother's kitchen. Man, that really was the Sweet Life.)

It's not exactly a new phrase, but as even the modest number of recipes in this chapter makes clear, there are a lot of fish in the sea: a lot of different tastes and textures, derived from a lot of different species of animals from a lot of different far-flung locations. (That's not surprising when you realize that water comprises 75 percent of the Earth's surface. The Pacific Ocean, the largest single geographic feature on Earth at more than 64 million square miles, occupies one-third of the planet. That's room for a lot of fish.) But what I've also tried to show with these recipes is that the variety of ways to prepare fish—seasoning, cooking, and serving—is virtually endless; certainly, it is limited only by your imagination.

In this chapter, as well as throughout this book, you'll find recipes using fish from fresh water and salt water, shellfish and scale fish, species from the Atlantic and Pacific Oceans. Of course whenever you cook fish it's far more important to go for what's freshest at your market rather than following the recipe to the letter; feel free to switch it up to take advantage of the daily catch. But whatever fish you choose. I hope you'll start with one that embodies the principles of sustainability. Pair it with just the right artisanal accompaniment—whether it's a single ripe cucumber or grits from South Carolina or a salad with just a drizzle of oil and maybe a squirt of citrus, and the result will be memorable.

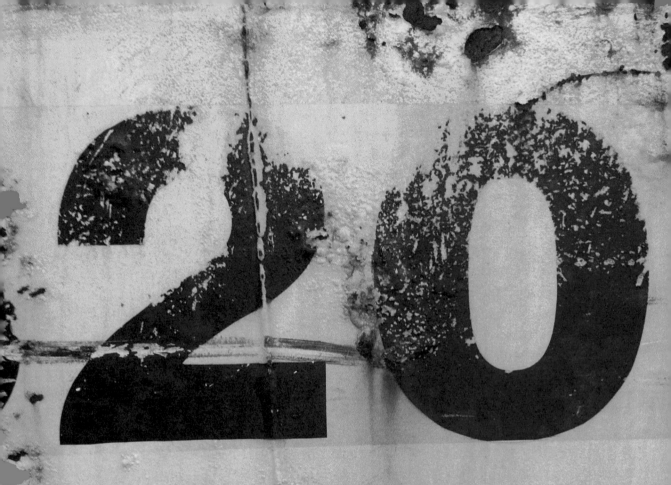

What I've tried to show with these recipes is that the variety of ways to prepare fish—seasoning, cooking, and serving—is virtually endless; certainly, it is limited only by your imagination.

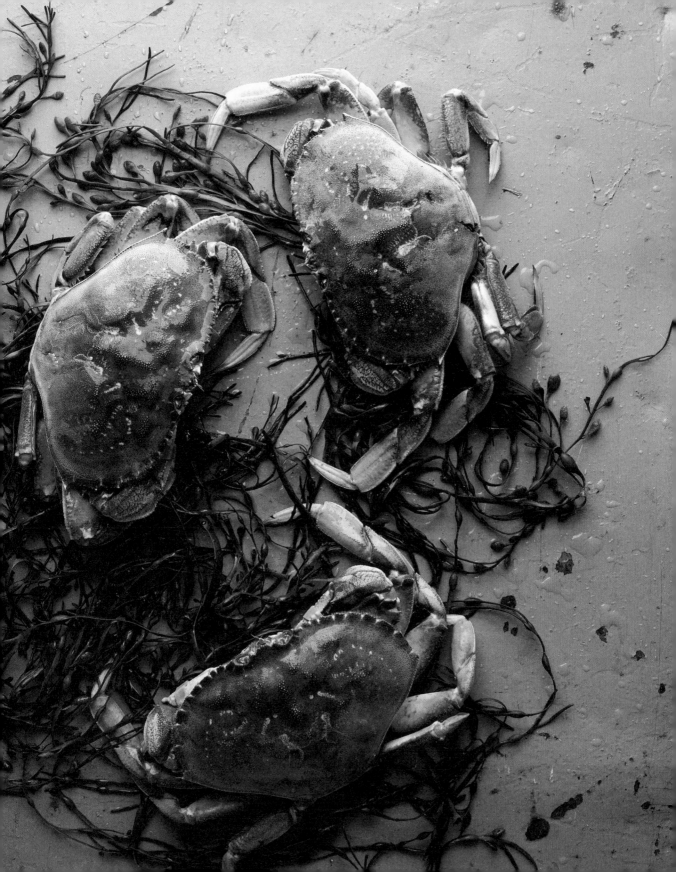

Steamed Little Neck Clams with Mustard Sauce

 As far back as I can remember, I have an image of my parents at the table, with heaping bowls of mussels or clams or shrimp in front of them, and lemon and butter everywhere, and they're sopping up every last drop of sauce with toasted bread, then washing it all down with a glass of white wine. This mustardy version is my take on that old family fave and it's like an insta-party. Mustard is one of the most widely used spices in the world, found in the cuisine of just about every culture. It is said to speed up metabolism, help lower blood pressure, and provide anti-inflammatory benefits. And it tastes so fine in this dish.

In a large skillet, heat the oil over medium-high heat. Add the fennel, onion, celery, mustard seeds, and coriander seeds and cook, stirring frequently, until the onion is translucent and the fennel starts to soften, 2 to 3 minutes.

Add the chili sauce, mustard, soy sauce, and vinegar and cook for 30 seconds to incorporate. Stir in the broth, clam juice, and Worcestershire sauce. Toss in the clams, cover the pan, and cook until the clams open, about 8 minutes. Discard any unopened shells.

Add the parsley and thyme to the pan and sprinkle with the lemon zest and juice, tossing well to combine. Season to taste with salt and pepper. Serve hot.

PER SERVING: 205 calories, 3 g protein, 17 g carbohydrates, 14 g total fat (2 g saturated), 0 mg cholesterol, 6 g fiber, 595 mg sodium

- ¼ cup olive oil
- 1 large fennel bulb, trimmed and cored, thinly sliced
- 1 large Vidalia or other sweet onion, thinly sliced
- 8 celery ribs, cut crosswise into ½-inch-wide pieces
- 1 tablespoon mustard seeds
- 1 teaspoon coriander seeds
- 2 tablespoons Thai sweet chili sauce
- 1 tablespoon Dijon mustard
- 2 tablespoons low-sodium soy sauce
- 2 tablespoons rice vinegar
- 2 cups low-sodium chicken broth
- ½ cup bottled clam juice
- 1 tablespoon Worcestershire sauce
- 2 pounds Little Neck clams, scrubbed
- ¼ cup flat-leaf parsley
- 3 tablespoons fresh thyme

  Grated zest and juice of 1 lemon

  Salt and freshly ground black pepper

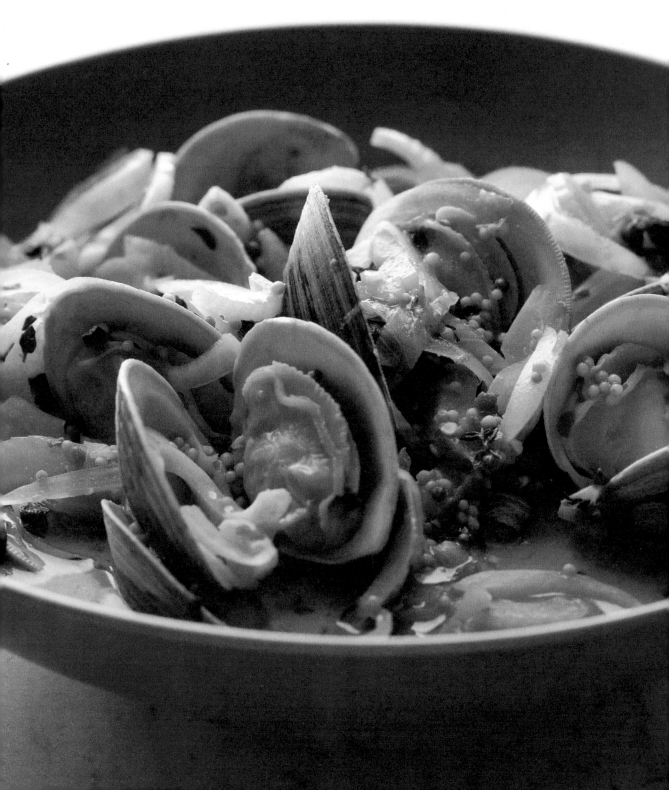

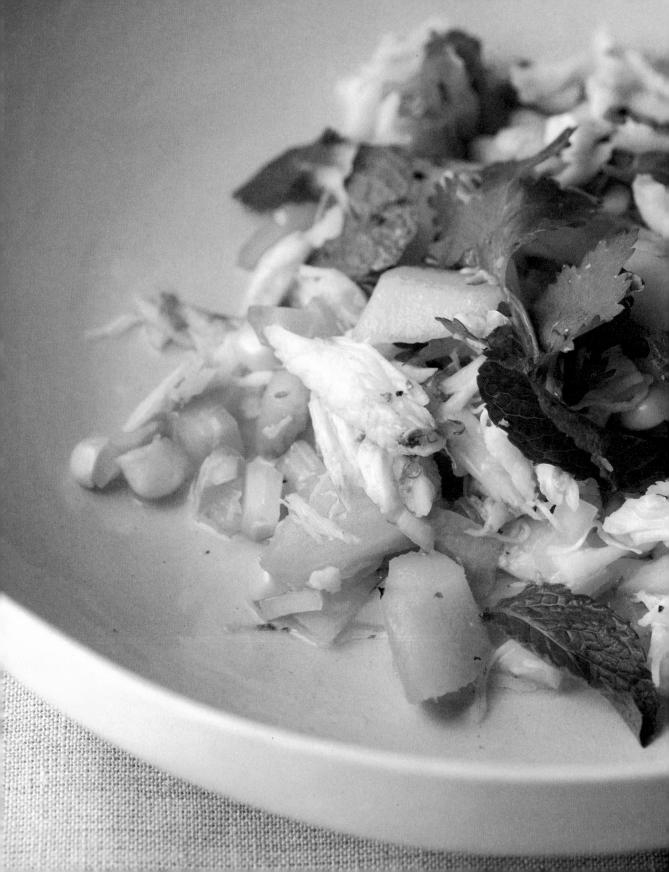

Peekytoe Crab Salad with Summer Corn

Summer. Summer. Summer. Summer. Get it? You need this in summer. Just like we need summer for our inner sanity, you need to eat this to channel the Sweet Life all summer long. You've heard of staples of the seasons? Meet summer's staple. Awesome flavors, bright colors, and oh so easy. I'm much more a fan of peekytoe or Jonah crab than, say, jumbo lump, which can be not only bland but triple the price as well. So you're welcome and you're welcome. If you can't get peekytoe, feel free to use lump, backfin, or jumbo lump crabmeat instead—anything sold fresh at the fish counter; leave the canned stuff on the shelf.

Dump the crabmeat into a mixing bowl and pick through for any pieces of shell or cartilage. Add the cucumber, mango, corn, mint, cilantro, lime zest and juice, and oil. Mix well with a rubber spatula taking care not to break up the crabmeat too much. Season to taste with salt and pepper.

PER SERVING: 377 calories, 43 g protein, 21 g carbohydrates, 13 g total fat (2 g saturated), 180 mg cholesterol, 3 g fiber, 652 mg sodium

1½ **pounds fresh peekytoe crabmeat or other fresh crabmeat**

1 **hothouse cucumber, peeled and finely chopped**

1 **mango, cut into small dice**

1 **cup corn kernels (2 or 3 ears)**

½ **cup loosely packed mint leaves**

½ **cup loosely packed cilantro leaves**

Grated zest and juice of 3 limes

3 **tablespoons Roasted Garlic Oil (page 93)**

Salt and freshly ground black pepper

Marinated Seared Scallops with Pecans and Okra Gumbo

Louisiana's got some serious mojo, and there's no dish that makes better use of that than gumbo. But the standard versions are downright heavy. Swapping out the usual over-cooked shrimp for quickly seared scallops makes the dish notably lighter and more modern. Sea scallops are an excellent source of vitamin B12, which helps in the formation of red blood cells and speeds the metabolism of carbohydrates, fats, and protein.

In a medium bowl, combine the Old Bay seasoning, chili powder, and 2 tablespoons of the oil. Add the scallops, stir to coat in the mixture, and set aside to marinate at room temperature for 30 minutes.

In a large nonstick skillet, heat 1 tablespoon of the oil over medium-high heat. Sear the scallops until they are golden brown, about 2 minutes on each side. Set aside.

In a large soup pot, heat the remaining ¼ cup oil over medium heat. Add the onion, garlic, bell peppers, ginger, and sausage. Cook, stirring frequently, until the onion is translucent and the sausage begins to brown, 3 to 4 minutes. Sprinkle in the flour and cook, stirring constantly, until the roux thickens and begins to turn golden brown, 6 to 7 minutes.

Stir in the tomato paste and wine and cook for 1 minute. Add the celery, okra, pecans, vinegar, Worcestershire sauce, crushed tomatoes, and broth. Bring the gumbo to a boil, reduce the heat to low, and simmer uncovered, stirring occasionally, for 1 hour 15 minutes. Adjust the seasonings to taste and stir in the scallions and parsley just before serving.

Spoon the gumbo into individual soup bowls and add 3 scallops per serving.

PER SERVING: 688 calories, 23 g protein, 35 g carbohydrates, 51 g total fat (10 g saturated), 56 mg cholesterol, 10 g fiber, 1,682 mg sodium

- 1 tablespoon Old Bay seasoning
- 1 teaspoon chili powder
- 3 tablespoons plus ¼ cup olive oil
- 1 dozen large sea scallops,
- 1 large yellow onion, finely diced
- 8 garlic cloves, finely chopped
- 2 red bell peppers, diced
- 2 tablespoons grated ginger
- 1 pound smoked sausage, sliced
- ¼ cup whole wheat flour
- ¼ cup tomato paste
- ½ cup dry white wine
- 4 celery ribs, thinly diced
- 1 pound fresh okra, sliced
- 1 cup chopped pecans
- 2 tablespoons balsamic vinegar
- 2 tablespoons Worcestershire sauce
- 1 can (28 ounces) crushed San Marzano tomatoes
- 4 cups low-sodium chicken broth
- 1 bunch scallions, thinly sliced
- ¼ cup chopped flat-leaf parsley

Pacific Cod with Clam Broth and Mustard Greens

When I was working at my first gig in New York City, I was obsessed with surfing the Internet for articles about other chefs and what they had on their menus. One night I was looking at the online menu for Luques, an LA restaurant owned by Suzanne Goin. There was a picture of some sort of fish with a roasted clam broth; and I thought it looked stellar. So I did some experimenting and came up with my own version. It's hearty enough to seem heavy but is actually quite the opposite—and easy on the stomach.

Preheat the oven to 375°F.

In a large soup pot, heat the butter and 2 tablespoons of the garlic oil over medium-high heat. Once the oil begins to shimmer and the butter starts to pop, add the onion, garlic, ginger, lemongrass, and mustard seeds. Cook, stirring frequently, until the onion is translucent, 2 to 3 minutes. Add the vinegar and wine and cook for 1 minute, scraping up any browned bits from the bottom of the pan to deglaze it.

Add the broth, jalapeño, mustard, Worcestershire sauce, lime zest and juice, and mustard greens. Bring the mixture to a boil, reduce the heat to medium-low, and add the clams. Cover the pot and cook until the clams open, 4 to 6 minutes. Discard any unopened shells. Stir in the parsley.

Season both sides of the cod fillets generously with salt and black pepper. In an ovenproof nonstick skillet, heat the remaining 1 tablespoon garlic oil over medium-high heat. Add the fish and cook for 2 minutes on one side, then flip for just a kiss on the other side. Flip the fish once more, transfer the pan to the oven and bake until the center is opaque and the fish flakes easily with a fork, about 7 minutes.

To serve, divide the clam broth among 4 shallow bowls and top with a fish fillet. Season to taste with salt and serve with the lemon wedges.

PER SERVING: 409 calories, 45 g protein, 17 g carbohydrates, 16 g total fat (4 g saturated), 108 mg cholesterol, 3 g fiber, 634 mg sodium

- 1 tablespoon unsalted butter
- 3 tablespoons Roasted Garlic Oil (page 93)
- 1 large yellow onion, diced
- 4 garlic cloves, finely chopped
- ¼ cup grated ginger
- ¼ cup chopped fresh lemongrass
- 1 teaspoon mustard seeds
- ⅓ cup rice vinegar
- ⅓ cup rice wine
- 3 cups low-sodium chicken broth
- 1 jalapeño chile pepper, diced
- 1 tablespoon Dijon mustard
- 1 tablespoon Worcestershire sauce
- Grated zest and juice of 2 limes
- 1 small bunch mustard greens, coarsely chopped
- 3 dozen Little Neck clams, scrubbed
- ½ cup chopped flat-leaf parsley
- 4 6-ounce cod fillets
- Salt and freshly ground black pepper
- 1 lemon, cut into 4 wedges

Squid with White Sesame Seeds and Jalapeño Peppers

Sautéed squid can be so elegant if cooked with precision. I'm not talking about mad-scientist precision, either—just a careful eye. Squid can turn into the kind of deep-fried rubber bands they sell at overcrowded street fairs in Little Italy in a heartbeat, so you have to be careful not to overcook it. It is usually fully cooked in less than a minute. It's meant to be soft and moist, not rubbery and bendable. The toasted sesame offers bits of texture, and the jalapeño provides some heat.

In a large skillet, heat the garlic oil over medium-high heat. Add the onion, bell pepper, jalapeños, garlic, sesame seeds, and coriander seeds and cook, stirring frequently, until the onion is translucent, 2 to 3 minutes. Pour in the wine and cook for 1 minute.

Add the squid and cook, stirring constantly, until the squid is coated in the mixture and heated through, 1 to 2 minutes. Add the cucumber, parsley, orange juice, and agave nectar. Cook for 1 to 2 minutes to heat through and marry the flavors.

Remove the pan from the heat and season to taste with salt and pepper. Serve hot.

PER SERVING: 252 calories, 25 g protein, 13 g carbohydrates, 11 g total fat (2 g saturated), 352 mg cholesterol, 1 g fiber, 81 mg sodium

- 3 tablespoons Roasted Garlic Oil (page 93)
- ½ large red onion, diced
- 1 red bell pepper, diced
- 1½ jalapeño chile peppers, seeded and finely chopped
- 3 garlic cloves, smashed and finely chopped
- 2 tablespoons white sesame seeds
- 1 teaspoon coriander seeds
- 2 tablespoons dry white wine
- 2 pounds squid, cleaned and cut into ¼-inch-wide rings, tentacles left whole
- 1 hothouse cucumber, finely diced
- ¼ cup chopped flat-leaf parsley
- Juice of ½ orange
- 1 tablespoon agave nectar
- Salt and freshly ground black pepper

Squid with Cherries, Tomatoes, Basil, and Mint

 6

There are so many health benefits to eating squid it's hard to know where to begin. Let's just say they are good for you from the inside (they're heart-healthy, they boost the immune system, and they help build teeth and bones) to the outside (great for the skin, hair, and nails). For diabetics in particular, eating these marine cephalopods may help stabilize sugar levels due to their rich supply of vitamin B3. I love squid, and this dish goes crazy with a diversity of tastes and textures.

Place the squid in a large bowl, add the milk, then cover the bowl tightly with plastic wrap and let the squid soak in the refrigerator overnight.

In a medium skillet, heat the garlic oil over medium-high heat. Add the onion, ginger, and garlic and cook, stirring frequently, until the onions are translucent, 2 to 3 minutes. Drain the squid (discard the milk mixture) and add to the pan, along with the cherries and blackening seasoning. Cook for 45 seconds without stirring, toss the pan a few times, then cook for another 30 seconds without stirring, or until the squid is just cooked through.

Add the wine and fish sauce and use a wooden spoon to scrape up any browned bits from the bottom of the pan to deglaze it. Add the tomatoes, scallions, basil, mint, and lime juice. Season to taste with salt and pepper. Serve hot.

PER SERVING: 247 calories, 26 g protein, 17 g carbohydrates, 8 g total fat (2 g saturated), 354 mg cholesterol, 2 g fiber, 344 mg sodium

- 2 **pounds squid, cleaned and cut into ¼-inch-wide rings, tentacles left whole**
- 2 **quarts whole milk**
- 2 **tablespoons Roasted Garlic Oil (page 93)**
- 1 **large yellow onion, thinly sliced**
- 2 **tablespoons grated ginger**
- 2 **tablespoons finely chopped garlic**
- 1 **cup pitted and sliced fresh cherries**
- 2 **tablespoons blackening seasoning**
- ¼ **cup dry white wine**
- 1 **teaspoon fish sauce**
- 2 **medium tomatoes, seeded and diced**
- 2 **scallions, green parts only thinly sliced**
- ½ **cup shredded fresh basil leaves**
- ¼ **cup shredded fresh mint leaves**
- **Juice of 2 limes**
- **Salt and freshly ground black pepper**

Steamed Pacific Halibut with Pickled Coleslaw

 4

Like most fish, halibut is great for helping reduce blood pressure; it also may protect against arthritis and is said to promote healthy brain function. One of the best fish markets in the world is Seattle's Pike Place. You've probably seen pictures of the guys in the fish stalls passing salmon to one another by hurling them through the air. It's kind of the best thing ever to watch or better yet take part in. While there, I had a piece of steamed halibut with coleslaw on top. Genius!

In a large skillet, heat the oil over medium-high heat. Add the onion, garlic, celery seeds, and cumin and cook until the onion is translucent, 2 to 3 minutes. Add the vinegar to the pan, cook for 15 to 30 seconds, then remove the pan from the heat and transfer the mixture to a large bowl to cool to room temperature.

Once the mixture has cooled, add the cabbage, cucumber, carrot, cilantro, mayonnaise, agave nectar, and lemon zest and juice. Toss well to combine and season to taste with salt and pepper.

While the coleslaw mixture cools, bring 2 inches of water to a boil in a wok or large saucepan. Set a bamboo steamer in the pan, making sure the bottom of the steamer is just above, not touching, the water level. Season the fish liberally with salt and pepper. Place the fish in the steamer, cover, and steam the fish until the fillets are opaque in the center and flake easily with a fork, 8 to 10 minutes.

Divide the salad among 4 plates and top with 1 fish fillet per serving.

PER SERVING: 406 calories, 38 g protein, 19 g carbohydrates, 19 g total fat (3 g saturated), 58 mg cholesterol, 3 g fiber, 184 mg sodium

- 2 **tablespoons olive oil**
- 1 **large red onion, thinly sliced**
- 2 **garlic cloves, smashed and finely chopped**
- 1 **teaspoon celery seeds**
- 1 **teaspoon ground cumin**
- 3 **tablespoons white wine vinegar**
- ½ **head napa cabbage, shredded**
- 1 **cucumber, peeled and finely diced**
- 1 **carrot, finely diced**
- ¼ **cup chopped fresh cilantro**
- 3 **tablespoons mayonnaise**
- 2 **tablespoons agave nectar**

  Grated zest and juice of 1 lemon

  Salt and freshly ground black pepper
- 4 **halibut fillets (6 ounces each)**

Simple Black Bass with Kale and Kalamata Olives

A portion of kale has only 36 calories but provides 192 percent of your daily vitamin A needs, meaning this dish has massive health benefits even before we get to the fish! It truly is a simple dish, made the way we like it: the best ingredients possible left alone to bask in all their beauty. And this one is *muy facil*. I like it especially for the moms who need to cook something up quick because it takes all of 15 minutes from start to finish. Okay, maybe 15 for me, 25 for you, but 25 tops! Olives are a bit high in monounsaturated fats, but they offer a substantial amount of vitamin E and anti-inflammatory benefits. And if you can't get black bass, don't freak out. You can sub cod, striped bass, really any nice thick white fillet of fish.

Preheat the oven to 350°F.

In a medium ovenproof skillet, heat 2 tablespoons of the oil over medium-high heat. Season the bass generously with salt and black pepper. Place it skin-side-down in the skillet and cook until the skin is golden brown, about 2 minutes. Place the pan in the oven and bake until the fish flakes easily, 5 to 7 minutes.

Meanwhile, in another medium skillet, heat the remaining 2 tablespoons oil over medium-high heat. Add the garlic and shallots and cook, stirring frequently, until they are translucent, 2 to 3 minutes. Add the kale in handfuls, being careful not to crowd the pan, and cook, stirring frequently, until wilted, 1 to 2 minutes.

Add the vinegar and use a wooden spoon to scrape up any browned bits on the bottom of the pan to deglaze it. Add the broth, orange zest and juice, parsley, roasted pepper, and olives and cook for 2 minutes to warm through and marry the flavors. Season to taste with salt and black pepper.

To serve, spoon the kale mixture into 4 individual bowls and top each serving with 1 bass fillet.

- 4 tablespoons olive oil
- 4 skin-on black bass fillets (6 ounces each)
  Salt and freshly ground black pepper
- 2 garlic cloves, finely chopped
- 2 shallots, finely chopped
- 1 large bunch kale, stems discarded, coarsely chopped
- 2 tablespoons white wine vinegar
- ¼ cup low-sodium chicken broth
  Grated zest and juice of 1 orange
- ¼ cup hand-torn flat-leaf parsley
- ½ roasted red pepper, finely chopped
- ¼ cup chopped kalamata olives

PER SERVING: 413 calories, 37 g protein, 24 g carbohydrates, 20 g total fat (3 g saturated), 70 mg cholesterol, 4 g fiber, 402 mg sodium

Mahi-Mahi with Rémoulade

 Do you know about rémoulade? If not, you're going to thank me. There are endless variations; Down South we turn it red with curry, and I've tasted it with pickles, horseradish, anchovies, capers—you name it. My own rendition adds some things that may surprise you, and it is the perfect seafood accompaniment. But don't stop there; you'll want to slather it on a cheeseburger or a grilled chicken sandwich, use it as a dip for veggies, and lots more.

To make the rémoulade: In a medium bowl, combine the mayonnaise, yogurt, mustard, vinegar, hot sauce, celery, scallions, parsley, egg, mustard seeds, and capers. Mix with a rubber spatula until well combined. Cover the bowl with plastic wrap and refrigerate until serving time.

To cook the fish: Preheat an outdoor grill or a stovetop grill pan to medium-high heat.

Drizzle the mahi-mahi with the oil and sprinkle with three-quarters of the lemon zest and juice. Season generously with salt and pepper. Grill the mahi-mahi until it flakes easily with a fork, 3 to 4 minutes per side.

Transfer the grilled fish to a serving platter and sprinkle with the remaining zest and juice. Serve with the rémoulade.

PER SERVING: 408 calories, 36 g protein, 14 g carbohydrates, 24 g total fat (4 g saturated), 189 mg cholesterol, 3 g fiber, 635 mg sodium

RÉMOULADE

- ½ cup low-fat mayonnaise
- ½ cup low-fat plain yogurt
- 1 tablespoon Dijon mustard
- 1 tablespoon red wine vinegar
- ½ teaspoon hot sauce
- 1 celery rib, finely diced
- 3 scallions, thinly sliced
- 2 tablespoons chopped flat-leaf parsley
- 1 hard-boiled egg, coarsely chopped
- 1 tablespoon mustard seeds
- 2 teaspoons rinsed, chopped capers

FISH

- 4 pieces (6 to 8 ounces each) mahi-mahi fillet
- 3 tablespoons olive oil
- Grated zest and juice of 4 lemons
- Salt and freshly ground black pepper

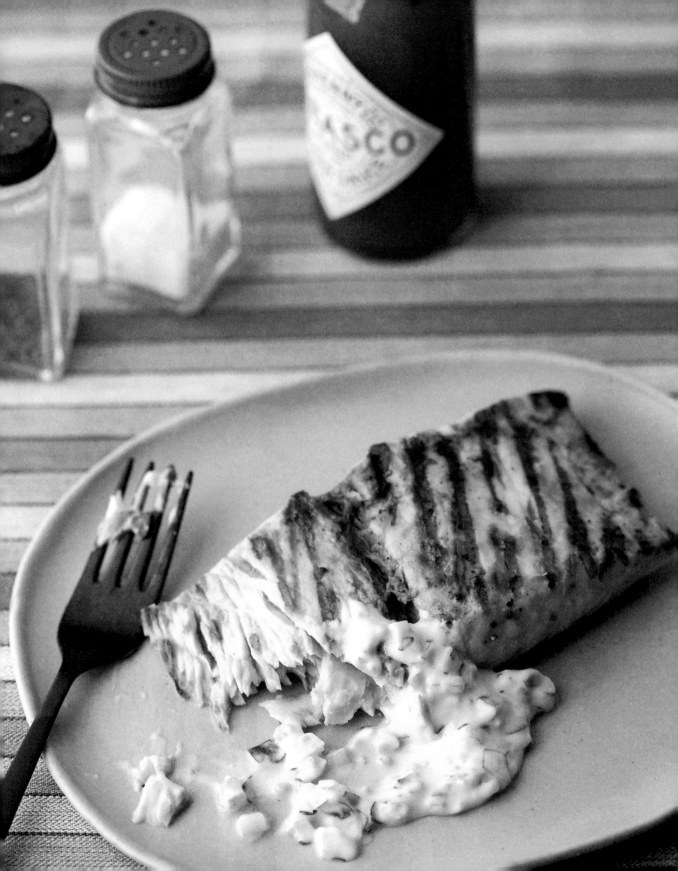

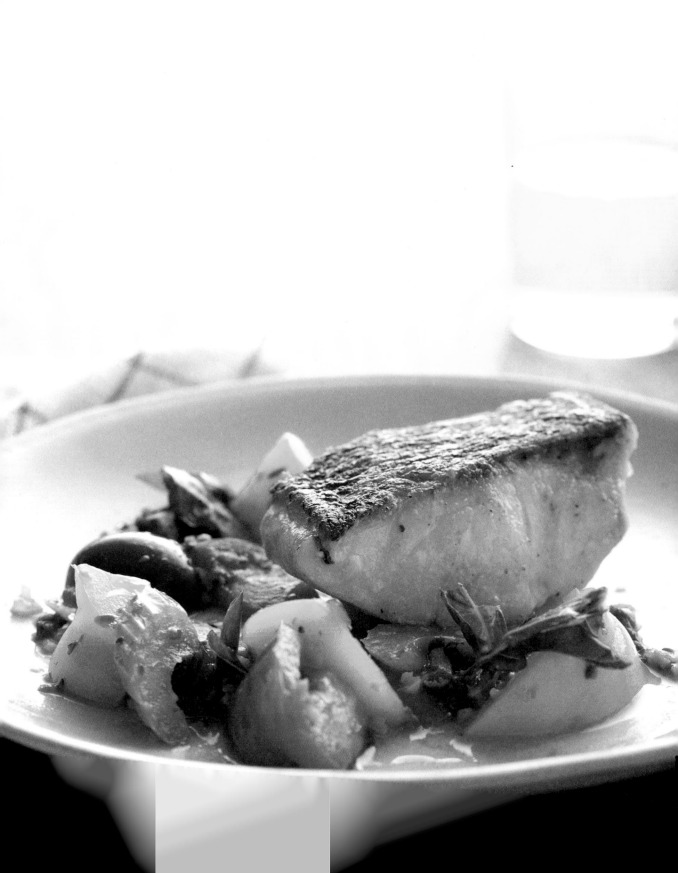

Striped Bass with Heirloom Tomato Scampi

 This one is Italy, pure and simple. Which is precisely what Italian cuisine is all about: Get yourself fresh, pure ingredients in season, plus some fine, real condiments and seasonings, and put it all together without a lot of fuss, and *ecco!* A simply superb meal, as healthy as they come and as good as eating gets. It's also beautiful on the plate. Note that scampi does not, in fact, mean shrimp, as many people think, but rather refers to the popular lemon, garlic, and oil preparation for shrimp in so many red-sauce Italian joints.

To cook the bass: Preheat the oven to 350°F.

In a large ovenproof nonstick skillet, heat the olive oil over medium-high heat. Season the fish liberally with salt and pepper and sprinkle with the lemon zest and juice. Once the oil begins to shimmer, place the fillets skin-side-down in the pan and let them cook, without moving them, until the skin is crisp and golden brown, 45 seconds to 1 minute. Give a light push to loosen the skin from the pan. Add the thyme sprigs to the pan. Transfer the pan to the oven and bake until the fish flakes easily with a fork, 6 to 8 minutes. Remove fish from the oven and transfer to paper towels.

To make the scampi: In a large skillet, heat the garlic oil over medium-high heat. Add the garlic, shallots, and fennel seeds and cook, stirring frequently, until the shallots are translucent, about 2 minutes. Add the celery and capers and cook until the celery has softened, about 2 minutes. Add the wine to the pan and cook until it is reduced by half, about 1 minute. Add the vinegar, lemon zest and juice, tomatoes, and basil and cook for 1 to 2 minutes to incorporate the flavors and heat the tomatoes through.

Serve the bass fillets topped with the tomato scampi.

PER SERVING: 424 calories, 35 g protein, 25 g carbohydrates, 21 g total fat (3 g saturated), 136 mg cholesterol, 7 g fiber, 252 mg sodium

BASS

- 2 tablespoons olive oil
- 4 striped bass fillets (6 ounces each)
- Salt and freshly ground black pepper
- Grated zest and juice of 1 lemon
- ½ bunch thyme sprigs

TOMATO SCAMPI

- 3 tablespoons Roasted Garlic Oil (page 93)
- 6 garlic cloves, finely chopped
- 2 shallots, finely diced
- 1 tablespoon fennel seeds, toasted in a dry skillet
- 4 celery ribs, sliced ¼ inch thick
- 1 tablespoon drained, chopped capers
- ¼ cup dry white wine
- 1 tablespoon red wine vinegar
- Grated zest and juice of 1 lemon
- 3 pounds mixed heirloom tomatoes, cut in wedges
- 1 cup tightly packed hand-torn fresh basil leaves

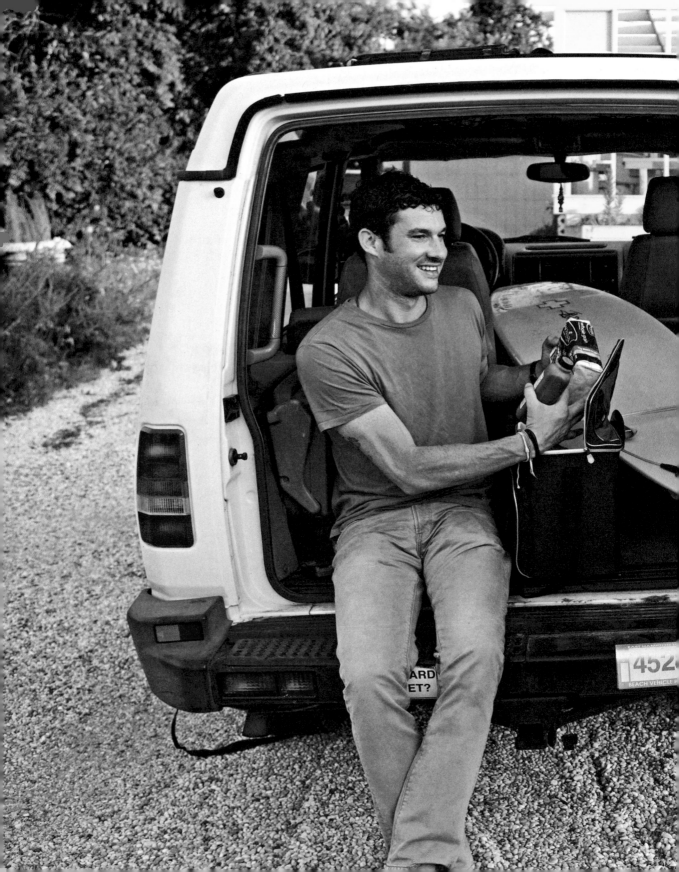

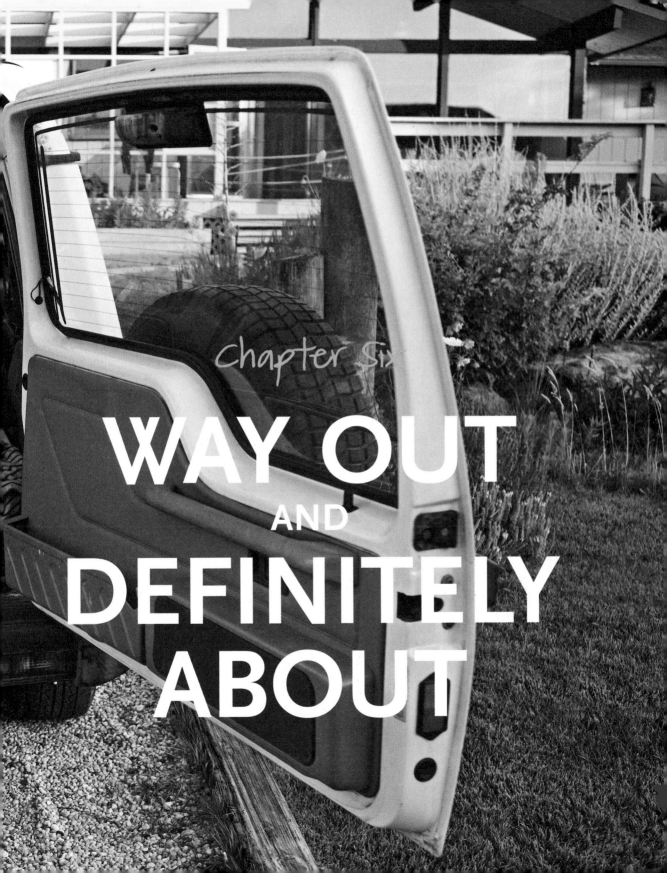

Chapter Six

WAY OUT
AND
DEFINITELY
ABOUT

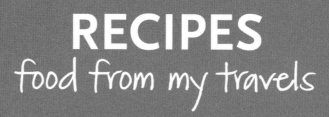

RECIPES
food from my travels

M ost people bring home souvenirs from their travels—fashions from Paris, glass objects from Venice, rugs from Istanbul. Me? Like most chefs, I bring home ideas for recipes, and in this chapter I'm offering a few of my travel-inspired recipes, plus some tips for making travel, whether cross-country, abroad, or a day trip to the farmers' market, a little less stressful.

As the saying goes, travel is broadening. Your senses are exposed to all sorts of new impressions, and as you absorb these sensations, your mind and imagination are stretched. Nowhere is this as true as with the sense of taste. Positive or negative, the sense-memory of a taste stays with you; it expands and, at least in my view, enriches your world of flavors.

As I write this, I'm remembering the first time I had udon, the thick wheat-flour noodles in broth that are a staple of the Japanese diet. It was a cold, cold morning in Tokyo, and the long flight and shift in time zones had me awake early—too early for the sightseeing venues to be open. In fact, nothing seemed open, except for this little hole-in-the-wall place with a steady stream of briefcase-toting businessmen entering and leaving. The steam coming out of the place had a tempting smell, so in I went, figuring I could at least warm up. Since I spoke no Japanese, I aped what the suits in front of me were doing and after a bit I was handed a piping-hot bowl filled to the brim with noodles, topped with bits of scallion. It smelled both rich and lively, and from the first delicious slurp, I knew I had discovered something that, for a foodie like me, would be absolutely life changing. I had another bowl and walked out of the place totally stoked by the taste and all the ideas for new recipes that were whipping around in my brain.

I've had similar experiences in many other places on earth: discovering açai in Brazil; treating myself to authentic fish and chips in London—not exactly a diabetic's dish, but I tell myself it's a professional necessity to check out the local eats; and just about any meal in my ancestral home, Italy. Don't let the last name Talbot fool you; my ancestry is mostly Sicilian, and my family's home of origin is quite simply a food lover's paradise—hard-core food porn. Once in Rome, down some side street I'll never find again, I stumbled into a place that was half living room, half kitchen. In the kitchen area were three women—sisters, I think, and all in their 70s—and they were cooking and washing dishes as if they were in their own home, which they were. They served me a grilled pork chop and peas—basically, the simplest of meals—and I actually laughed out loud as I ate it because it was the best damned pork chop and peas I had ever eaten. I've carried the memory of it for years, and it has influenced countless recipes I've created as a professional chef.

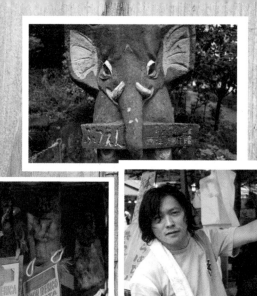
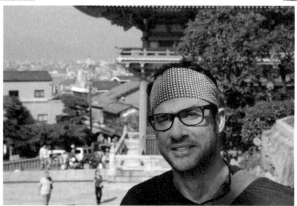
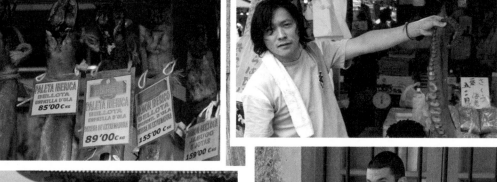
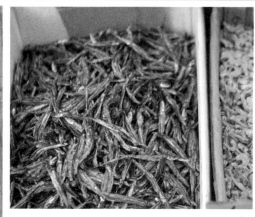
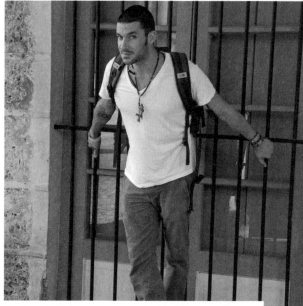
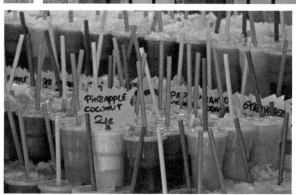

THE DIABETIC TRAVELER

When I was about 25, I decided to find out firsthand if, as a diabetic, I could travel on my own, explore a different culture, and cook different kinds of food. So I packed up my backpack with a week's worth of underwear, my chef's coat, combat boots, a hoodie, and of course lots of insulin, blood meters, and syringes—along with loads of Lifesavers and juice—and headed for Paris, the food lover's Mecca. The experiment taught me that I *could* travel solo as a diabetic, but it took some doing. Where travel is concerned, diabetics have to be particularly careful—we can do it, but we have to take particular precautions.

Actually, the dangers can come at you in funny ways—like the night in Tokyo when the door to my tiny hotel room was kicked in at 4:00 a.m. with an explosion of noise that shot me upright off my tatami mat, stopped my heart cold, and lit up the words "holy shit!" in neon in my brain. Eight guys with guns in one hand and nightsticks in the other stood there, weapons pointed, faces screaming incomprehensibly in Japanese. Instinctively I raised my hands—the classic don't-shoot gesture—and they reacted as if I had drawn a weapon, coming at me with the nightsticks pointed at my head. "Holy shit!" I blubbered it aloud this time, alternating it over and over and over with "holy Mary mother of God!" as their screaming grew louder.

If you've ever seen the classic movie *Midnight Express*, or watched *Return to Paradise* with Vince Vaughn and Joaquin Phoenix, you know the nightmare I'm talking about. Guns, nightsticks, the guys screaming in Japanese, me on the floor, cowering in my boxers, the rosary racing through my brain. It seemed to go on forever.

"We're from the Tokyo Organized Crime unit," the main guy finally said in English, "and we have reason to believe you're trafficking in illegal drugs. We take this crime very seriously in this country, and we're going to search your things. Stand up, but do not speak."

They rifled through my luggage. I thought how easy it would be for them to plant stuff on me and wondered briefly if Japanese courts had an appeals process.

Then they found my syringes—right there in my Dopp kit.

They talked among themselves, looked in the Dopp kit again, talked again. And suddenly I could feel that something in the atmosphere had shifted.

"Sick?" the main guy asked me.

I nodded vigorously. "Yes, yes," I said. "Diabetic. I have diabetes." I was still nodding. "I have insulin there, too. And blood meters. Test strips. For diabetes. I'm a diabetic."

The cops lowered their guns and backed out of the tiny room. Just before closing the door, the main guy turned and looked at me. "At least you have a very special memory of being in Japan," he said.

Yeah, right.

But don't worry. If you're a diabetic who loves to travel, the risk that your supply of syringes will get you shot by narcs is far lower than the risk of feeling sick and having run out of syringes. That's the real danger, and it's why we diabetics need to get totally obsessive about precautions when we travel, building those precautions into a routine, and then rehearsing that routine until it becomes automatic. You need to think about any problem that might conceivably arise, from losing your luggage entirely to finding yourself hours away from the closest meal, and troubleshoot how you might deal with it. The aim is for these safeguards and habits to become so instinctive that you shift into gear like a robot, so that you really can let your wanderlust run wild—unrestrained and unrestricted. Of course I can't *always* predict every bump in the road that might present itself, detail-obsessed though I typically am.

On a recent trip to Alaska I missed one tiny thing—and almost got put through a real wringer. I was in our 49th state to raise diabetes awareness. A much-needed trip because, sadly, diabetes is rampant there. The far-flung native villages in particular are hotbeds of the disease. The traditional way of life—hunting for whales and seals and caribou—has become a part-time endeavor now, so the native people have had to change their way of eating. But in place of the ancient traditions have come processed food, sodas, candy bars, boxed breads, canned meats, and poorly frozen vegetables; the villages are just too distant and too hard to reach for much else. The result is that Alaska has a heaping portion of type 2 diabetes and an increasing incidence of type 1 diabetes.

I was on a tiny seaplane heading back to Anchorage from a remote wilderness location, and we were being buffeted like a paper airplane lost in the atmosphere. Up, down, left, right: Anyone with a weak stomach or a fear of flying would have passed out by now, and anything not lashed down was floating around the cabin as if we were at zero G. Including my bottle of Humalog—the fast-acting insulin that is the essential tool for managing my disease; I do not leave home without it. Now, I watched helplessly as it shot out of my vest

Plane Eats

Airplane food blows. I don't care if you ordered the special kosher meal or are in the cockpit flying your own Gulfstream G6, the food is still going to suck; there's no way to do real cooking in a airplane galley at 37,000 feet. That's why homemade snacks are so important, and I've got a doozy I don't leave home without. I call it the Ninja Snack Pack in honor of those fabulous, black-costumed, badass characters I idolized when I was a little boy. They embodied cool, stoic, total energy, and the Ninja Snack Pack is something of the ultimate nutrition and energy feed. That's true for anyone anywhere, but it's especially true for diabetics.

Here's what I take:

Wasa crackers
Homemade peanut butter
Hummus
Tart apple wedges
Dried açai granola
Celery sticks

The cracker is a high-fiber, low-GI vehicle for getting the peanut butter and hummus up to your face and into your mouth. Peanut butter is the star player here: It is pure protein and will sustain you no matter where or how far you're going. Ditto for the hummus, which is a bit more luxurious and silky. Also, I'm addicted to hummus, so I pack it all the time.

By "tart" apples I mean apples quickly dipped in lemon juice and a touch of vinegar. Why? Well, as you've probably heard, an apple a day covers you for fruits and veggies, but once you cut into one, it gets brown and oxidized; the quick pickling dip stops all that. Plus, it brings out the natural flavor and sweetness of the apples.

As for the granola, yes, it's a bit higher in carbs than the other items in the Snack Pack

and should therefore be eaten sparingly just for the crunch and munch effect, not as a whole bowl or cup.

Celery is key. If you're not keeping up with your water intake while on the road—and sometimes it's hard to do—these pups, which are 80 percent water, can really help keep you lubed. So dig in and munch up.

If the mix in my Ninja Snack Pack is not to your liking, make your own, following this formula: It should be nonperishable and have nutritional value. It should also taste good to you. You want something that will tide you over so you arrive somewhat fueled up but not too filled up. What you *don't* want is to end up filling up on prepackaged, wilted fruit that has been dipped in sulfites to keep it looking fresh for days on end, or some sort of barbecued chicken wrap that was quick and easy to buy.

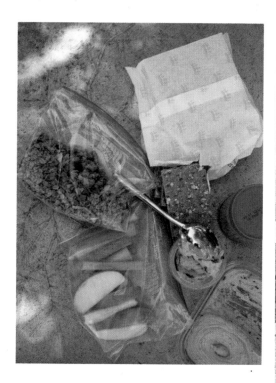

pocket, hit the ceiling, then smashed to the floor and broke into way too many pieces. It is not a good feeling to see your lifeline shatter and then seep away. In addition, have you ever smelled insulin? It is gnarly, and that's really all you want to know.

So the plane is tumbling through the air, the stench is nearly unbearable for me and everybody else on the plane, and we still have 45 more minutes of flying time.

And that's when I began to panic. I panicked because I was out of the stuff that keeps me healthy and was thus defenseless against my disease, because I was 10,000 feet up in the air and powerless to do anything about it, and because my friends on the trip with me were panicking on my behalf. For me, stress can do one of two things: send my blood sugar count plummeting or kick it in the ass and shoot it way up. In this particular case, it was up; I clocked it at 120 on the meter—a bit toward the high end of my 90-to-130-ish range, but still under the limit. *Forty-five minutes,* I said to myself. *Not so long. Try to chill.* That's all I could do. I smiled at my friends and faked it, because sometimes when you fake it, it works—as it did in this case—although there was nothing I could do about the smell.

The plane got us to Anchorage, and I made a few calls, headed for a pharmacy, and put that incident to rest. Up until that trip, I'd always been backup-ready for a drop in blood sugar but never for a burst to a high sugar count. If I hadn't forced myself to climb down from panic during those final 45 minutes till we landed in Anchorage, I could have been a very sick bloke indeed. Since that trip, wherever I go, I carry one bottle of insulin on me and anywhere from one to three bottles in a jacket or padded bag or something else that I carry. It's now just as much part of my travel preparations as grabbing my passport or packing a toothbrush.

DO YOUR HOMEWORK AT HOME

The routine has to start before you set foot out the door. Whether you're going overseas for a month or out of town for a weekend, the first thing to do is to check on the available medical facilities where you're going: pharmacies, doctors, clinics, hospitals. You also want to know how tough it will be to get to these facilities, and you want to be sure that there is cell phone service or a landline phone or Internet connection in case you need to summon help fast.

Nothing is easier than finding this stuff out. Not only can you Google it; you can Google Earth it and zoom in on the street view of the front door of a pharmacy 10,000 miles away. It means you know you're covered, and that's essential.

Next, gather your medical supplies for packing. On this score, there's an old saying that works for me: If you want to be sure you've got it, bring it with you. For just about any kind of travel where luggage gets checked and spends time away from you—plane, train, even bus—that means having what you need in your carry-on as well as in your checked luggage.

Make sure your carry-on has backup, too. (That's the step I forgot on that trip in Alaska, and it cost me.) I always make sure that my backup has backup, that it's on me as well as

Thai-In

You'll see a strong Thai influence in many of the dishes in this book. I love all the cuisines of the Far East, but I particularly love the cuisine of Thailand for its light touch and its freshness. Certainly Thai food can be spicy—you won't find anything hotter than street-food snacks in Bangkok, if you dare—but what really distinguishes this cuisine is the variety of its fresh spices and herbs and, I would add, the aromatic quality these spices and herbs bring to every dish. Lime and cilantro, basil and mint, ginger and lemongrass, as well as coconut milk, are all used enthusiastically, so that each dish, or at least each meal, provides a balance of taste sensations—sweet and sour, salty and spicy, and even a touch of bitter. It's this balance that gives Thai cuisine its special character, and when it all comes together in a dish like Steamed Thai Mussels (page 168), an easy one-pot meal that can be the centerpiece of any party, there's nothing better.

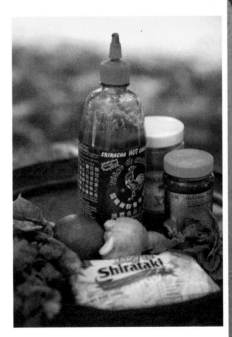

Other Asian ingredients I like to keep on hand for impromptu noodle dishes, to doctor up a vinaigrette, or slather on a burger, and a million other uses:

- **Toasted sesame oil**
- **Sesame seeds (pretoasted and ground)**
- **Sriracha and Asian chili paste (sambal oelek)**
- **Soba, udon, and shirataki noodles**
- **Bok choy**

in my luggage, and that it's wrapped in some safe and secure protective covering so it won't bend, break, shatter, spill, evaporate, or slip out of a hole in my backpack or suitcase.

Figuring out how much to bring isn't that tough. Basically, you just multiply your daily kit—the stuff you don't leave home without on a day-to-day basis—by the number of days you're going to be away. Then add an extra amount for contingency backup.

How much extra? The longer you'll be away and the more remote or exotic or new-to-you the place you're visiting, the more supplies you want to have on you. If I'm flying from New York to London for the weekend, that's a low-risk contingency. London is a huge world capital, has some of the best medical facilities in the world, is open around the clock, and I speak the language—sort of. But if I get an invitation to surf off Patagonia or heli-snowboard in the northern mountains of India or even do a cooking demo in a town in the middle of my own country that I know nothing about, I'll want to double-down on the extra supplies.

ROAD TRIP!

It's kind of the American Dream, isn't it? You're lighting out for the territory, a long stretch of highway ahead of you, windows down, elbow resting on the open window and catching the breeze. You can sing off-key as loud as you want along with the music or listen to a book you never got around to reading, and if you're on an interstate, you won't see a red light or a stop sign from sea to shining sea.

The problem for diabetics—again, it's a problem for everyone, but more serious for us—is the food available along the way. Interstate rest stops offer fast-food or sub-par chain restaurants. Period. If that's all you ate driving across country, you'd not only gain 20 pounds, you'd get sick. Eating that kind of processed food is like ingesting bricks. Your body doesn't know what to do with what it's taking in, so the stuff just sits there and clogs your system. Your skin breaks out, you get bloated, you feel absolutely terrible. I'm not kidding: This stuff is really dangerous. It's what's turning so much of our population into a heart attack waiting to happen. And on the road, unfortunately, it's hard to find other choices.

There's a solution, and all it takes is some room in the trunk or the backseat or the cargo area. Plus, you'll need to invest in a cooler and a bunch of those eco-friendly reusable grocery bags. And here's another useful tip: I always bring a small wooden cutting board, Handi Wipes, some disposable flatware and plates—try the eco-friendly kind made from potato starch—and a roll of paper towels.

This is the solution: Even if you have to drive 20 miles off the interstate to find real food, fill the bags, and fill the cooler. You want the basics—quick snack foods as well as some fresh fruit and vegetables and the odds and ends that can match your different food cravings and moods.

My typical practice is to fill the bags with trail mix, baked string bean chips, canned tuna, canned peas, and some sort of sea-salted toasted seeds. I toss fruit, sliced deli turkey, pickles, cheese, a head of iceberg lettuce, prepared deli egg salad, brown rice, marinated or spicy tofu, baby carrots, cucumbers, and ranch dressing, and mayo in a cooler. (Ranch dressing? Mayo? No, these aren't really healthy or diabetic-friendly, but they *are* the two best single creations of mankind as far as this chef is concerned. Everything in moderation, right? And sometimes you just have to put your hand in the cookie jar.)

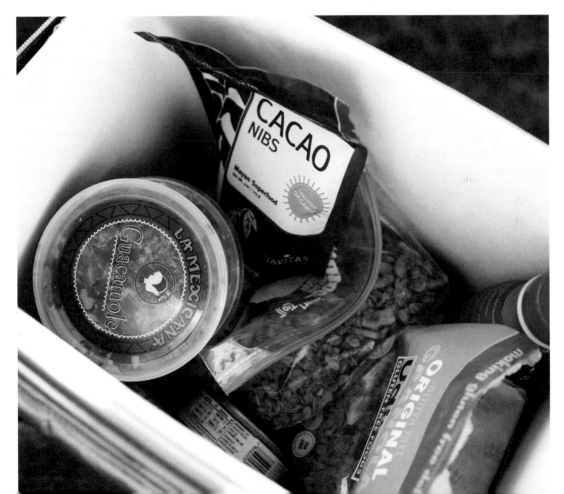

I also keep a 10-pack of Nantucket Nectars in the car at all times, putting one or two at a time into the cooler.

When I start to feel peckish, I pull over, open up a can of tuna and a can of peas, mix them together—I know it sounds gross, but my mother made it up, and it has been my weird fave food since I was a kid—and chow down.

And if there's a hot lady with me, we'll find some back road, set out the disposable flatware and plates, fix up a salad of lettuce, cukes, and carrots—yes, with ranch dressing—and some deli meat or tofu or both, open a bottle of wine and watch the sunset, then cozy up for a night's sleep in the backseat, and that makes for a very good cross-country drive.

LOCAVORES ON THE ROAD

One of the best things about travel lately is that when you make that 20-mile detour off the interstate, you have a good chance of finding a farmers' market with a spread of just-harvested, local food from the surrounding area. There are more and more of these every day everywhere. You know what went up in 2008 when everything else in the economy went down? Cookbook sales and the number of farmers' markets popping up in neighborhoods near you. Why? People want value for money, and they want to be connected to the food they eat. They're right. Remember that you are 100 percent what you eat. When you eat fresh and local and as close to the source of the food as possible, you're simply getting food that is simply better tasting and better for you. It is also a totally great way to save money—you cut out the middleman—and contribute to sustainable agriculture. I don't know about you, but all of that is pretty appealing to me.

And now you can eat local all over the world. It's as easy as asking a reputable hotel concierge for details or logging on for a basic Google search. Try searching for "farmers' markets Paris." You'll bring up a hell of a lot of references—a great starting point for getting to local websites or food blogs quickly and then navigating easily to what you're looking for.

Once you find a market you want to explore, go early. Always. The earlier the better. Why? For the same reason it pays to go surfing at first light: It's just you—and maybe your friends—and you get first dibs on everything; the place belongs to you. Everybody else is on their way to work or still sleeping, and you're out there getting to choose among the primo vegetables of that day's harvest, the freshest loaf of bread, the first *tranche* of cheese or meat.

Unless you're in a cooler-equipped car, my suggestion is to buy only what you are going to eat that day. If you're overseas, remember that if you buy liquids like oil and vinegar or jellies and honey and the like, you're going to have to finish it all or leave it behind when you board the plane for home—unless you are buying sealed bottles and jars to pack in your checked luggage. (In which case, be careful: A cracked bottle of olive oil or broken honey jar can create mayhem in a suitcase.) Instead, think picnic and feast on what you've purchased right then and there as you enjoy the show: Local markets are legendary for people-watching. Are there better reasons for travel than these two—seeing how other people live and eating what they eat? I don't know if I would dub the recipes in this chapter "wild," but they're going to bring out the *Top Chef* in you. You'll be finding, marinating, and searing exotic ingredients like harissa, putting together foods you never thought you'd put together—and going for the Big Haute Cuisine Moment. Try these recipes and I think you'll agree with me: There's nothing better in the world.

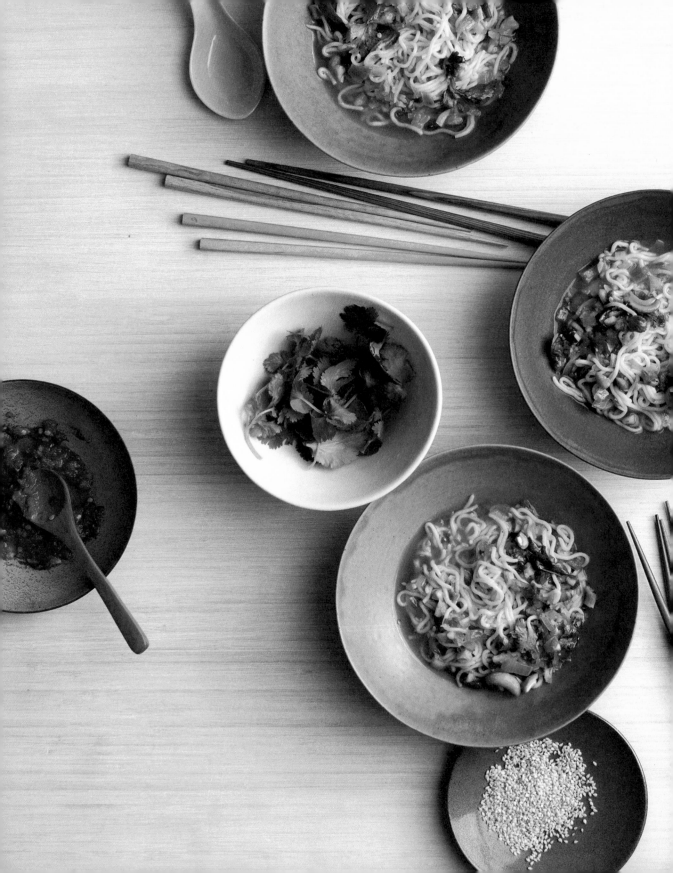

Shirataki Noodles with Cashews and Chiles

4

I have an appreciation of udon noodles that borders on obsession, but when I want to go lighter on the carbs, shirataki noodles are a nice, low-carb alternative. Because they are made from tofu and yam flour, they have minimal carbs. You can make this dish on the fly too, when you're in a rush. It's clean, light, and well balanced. I stock up on shirataki in Japanese markets around New York, and they are widely available in health food stores and some large supermarkets.

Rinse the noodles under cold running water and drain well, then transfer them to a large bowl and toss with 1 tablespoon of the sesame oil to keep them from sticking together.

In a large skillet, heat the remaining 2 tablespoons sesame oil over medium-high heat. Add the onion, garlic, ginger, jalapeños, and sesame seeds and cook, stirring frequently, until the onions are translucent and aromatic, 2 to 3 minutes. Add the vinegar, agave nectar, and chili paste, stirring well to combine. Mix in the broth, cashews, cilantro, and soy sauce and cook for 1 to 2 minutes to marry the flavors.

Pour the sauce over the noodles. Let the noodles rest in the sauce for a couple of minutes before serving.

PER SERVING: 227 calories, 4 g protein, 19 g carbohydrates, 16 g total fat (2 g saturated), 0 mg cholesterol, 2 g fiber, 448 mg sodium

- 2 packages (16 ounces total) tofu shirataki noodles
- 3 tablespoons toasted sesame oil
- 1 large red onion, diced
- 4 garlic cloves, finely chopped
- 2 tablespoons finely chopped fresh ginger
- 2 fresh jalapeño chile peppers, seeded and finely chopped
- 2 tablespoons sesame seeds, toasted in a dry skillet
- 2 tablespoons rice vinegar
- 2 tablespoons agave nectar
- 1 teaspoon sambal oelek chili paste
- 1 cup low-sodium chicken broth
- ¼ cup chopped cashews
- ⅓ cup hand-torn fresh cilantro
- 2 tablespoons low-sodium soy sauce

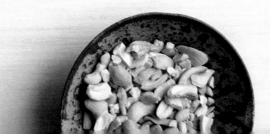

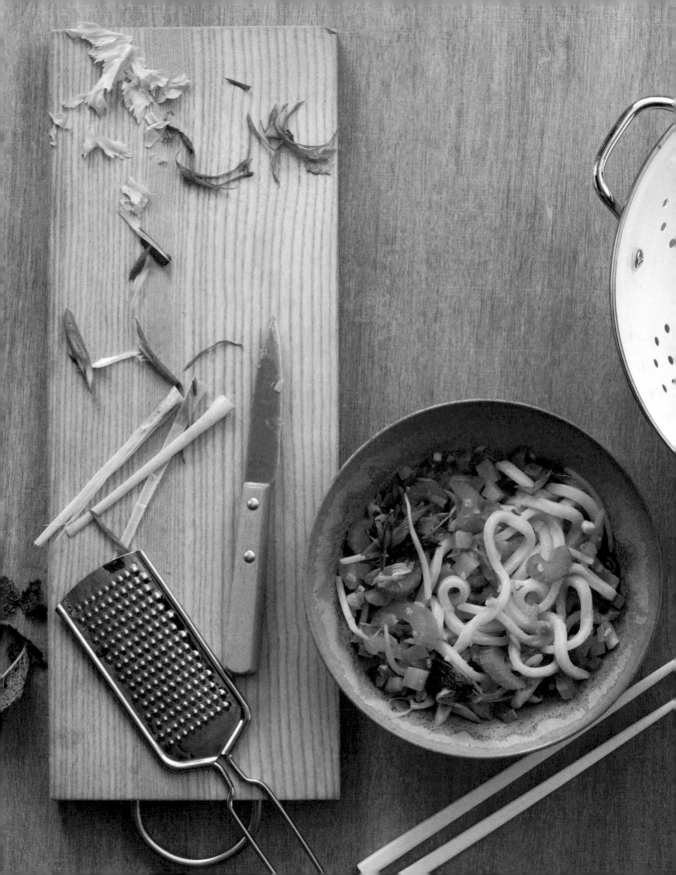

Shirataki Noodles with Spicy Scallions, Bean Sprouts, and Mint

 Udon noodles are typically served in a crystal-clear dashi broth, the seaweed and fish stock basic to Japanese cuisine, and topped off with fresh scallions and *togarashi*, Japan's hot-hot chili pepper condiment. A bowl of shirataki noodles is much like udon but with few carbs and is the perfect closer to a day of going from one shrine or temple site to another in Japan, or to a day of errands and meetings in New York, or any time at all.

Bring a large pot of salted water to a boil. Add the noodles and cook for a minute or 2 to warm through. Drain the noodles and set aside.

In a large skillet, heat the sesame oil over medium-high heat. Add the garlic, ginger, lemongrass, celery, onion, shallot, carrots, and vinegar and cook until the onion is translucent and the mixture is fragrant, 2 to 3 minutes. Add the broth, bean sprouts, scallions, mint, and chili paste and cook for another 2 minutes. Add the drained noodles and cook for 1 minute, tossing with tongs to combine.

Divide the noodles among 6 bowls. Season each serving to taste with salt and pepper and sprinkle with lime zest and juice. Serve hot.

PER SERVING: 107 calories, 3 g protein, 16 g carbohydrates, 5 g total fat
(1 g saturated), 0 mg cholesterol, 3 g fiber, 118 mg sodium

2 8-ounce packages tofu shirataki noodles

2 tablespoons toasted sesame oil

6 garlic cloves, finely chopped

¼ cup finely grated fresh ginger

2 tablespoons finely chopped fresh lemongrass

4 celery ribs, thinly sliced on the diagonal

1 large red onion, diced

1 shallot, diced

2 carrots, diced

2 tablespoons rice vinegar

1 cup low-sodium chicken broth

1 cup bean sprouts, coarse stems discarded

3 scallions, thinly sliced on the diagonal

¼ cup chopped fresh mint leaves

1 tablespoon sambal oelek chili paste

Salt and freshly ground black pepper

Grated zest and juice of 2 limes

Shirataki Noodles with Parsnips, Chili Paste, and Mint

6 If you're looking for an easy, meatless entrée, you'll be very happy with this, but it's easy to adapt if you want to add some protein. Fresh seafood works wonderfully with the clean, crisp flavors of the parsnip and mint, so there are a lot of things you could try here and come out happy. A few years back I had this on a restaurant menu and we sometimes added seared scallops or even razor clams, which were phenomenal.

Bring a large pot of water to a boil. Add the noodles and boil for a minute or so to heat through. Drain well and set aside.

In a large skillet, heat the garlic oil and sesame oil over medium heat. Add the parsnips, ginger, and Roasted Garlic and cook until the parsnips are fork-tender, 2 to 3 minutes. Increase the heat to medium-high and add the tahini, chili paste, broth, cider, and vinegar. Cook for 2 minutes to heat through and marry the flavors

Add the mint and the noodles and toss with tongs to combine. Season to taste with salt and pepper. Sprinkle with the orange zest and juice and toss again.

PER SERVING: 164 calories, 2 g protein, 13 g carbohydrates, 13 g total fat (2 g saturated), 1 mg cholesterol, 2 g fiber, 52 mg sodium

- 2 **8-ounce packages tofu shirataki noodles**
- 2 **tablespoons Roasted Garlic Oil (page 93)**
- 2 **tablespoons toasted sesame oil**
- 1 **cup peeled, chopped parsnips**
- 2 **tablespoons finely chopped fresh ginger**
- 12 **cloves Roasted Garlic (page 93), lightly mashed**
- 2 **tablespoons tahini**
- 1 **tablespoon chili paste**
- ¼ **cup low-sodium chicken broth**
- 2 **tablespoons organic apple cider or apple juice**
- 2 **tablespoons cider vinegar**
- 1 **cup hand-torn fresh mint leaves**

  Salt and freshly ground black pepper

  Grated zest and juice of 1 orange

Coconut and Lemongrass Soup with Lime and Cilantro

 The food of Thailand has always been, and will continue to be, one of my favorite cuisines. It also happens to be my take-out favorite. But I love to play around with these flavors when I cook for myself too, like in this easy, light version of tom ka gai, a traditional soup I can't get enough of. I go heavy on the lemongrass; for me, the more the merrier.

In a medium soup pot, heat the oil over medium heat. Add the onion, lemongrass, ginger, jalapeños, and garlic and cook until the onion is translucent and the garlic and ginger have softened, about 2 minutes.

Mix in the broth, coconut milk, and agave nectar. Increase the heat to high and bring the mixture to a boil. Reduce to a simmer and cook, uncovered, for 30 minutes.

Add the bean sprouts, cilantro, and lemon zest and juice. Cook for 2 minutes to marry the flavors. Serve hot.

PER SERVING: 402 calories, 7 g protein, 24 g carbohydrates, 35 g total fat (22 g saturated), 0 mg cholesterol, 3 g fiber, 298 mg sodium

- 3 tablespoons Roasted Garlic Oil (page 93)
- 1 small red onion, thinly sliced
- ¼ cup finely chopped fresh lemongrass
- ¼ cup finely chopped fresh ginger
- 2 jalapeño chile peppers, seeded and diced
- 3 garlic cloves, smashed and finely chopped
- 2 cups low-sodium chicken broth
- 2 cups light coconut milk
- 2 tablespoons agave nectar
- 1 cup bean sprouts
- ¼ cup chopped fresh cilantro
- Grated zest and juice of 2 limes

Steamed Thai Mussels

 4

Quintessentially Thai and quintessentially mussels—and that's the point. This dish is consistently one of the top sellers at The Surf Lodge, and it's as simple as it is popular. A variety of spices and herbs plays with the taste and add the dimension of aroma—and what it all does is bring out the inherent goodness and cleanliness and health and flavor of fresh, steamed mussels. To my mind it's the perfect way to eat.

In a large saucepan, heat the butter and oil over medium heat. Once the butter has melted, toss in the garlic, ginger, shallot, and lemongrass and cook, stirring frequently, until the shallot is translucent and the garlic and ginger have softened, 2 to 3 minutes.

Add the mussels to the pan, pour in the wine, and cook for 1 minute. Add the soy sauce, fish sauce, and pepper flakes and simmer for 1 minute. Stir in the coconut milk and lime juice, cover the pan, and steam the mussels until they are open, about 2 minutes. Discard any unopened shells.

Season the broth to taste with salt and black pepper, stir in the cilantro, and serve hot.

PER SERVING: 356 calories, 22 g protein, 17 g carbohydrates, 23 g total fat (11 g saturated), 63 mg cholesterol, 1 g fiber, 857 mg sodium

- **2 tablespoons unsalted butter**
- **2 tablespoons olive oil**
- **2 tablespoons smashed and finely chopped garlic**
- **2 tablespoons finely chopped fresh ginger**
- **1 shallot, finely chopped**
- **2 tablespoons chopped fresh lemongrass**
- **1 to 1½ pounds mussels, scrubbed, debearded, and rinsed**
- **⅓ cup dry white wine**
- **1 tablespoon low-sodium soy sauce**
- **1 teaspoon fish sauce**
- **1 teaspoon red pepper flakes**
- **½ cup coconut milk**
- **Juice of 1 lime**
- **Salt and freshly ground black pepper**
- **½ bunch fresh cilantro, hand torn**

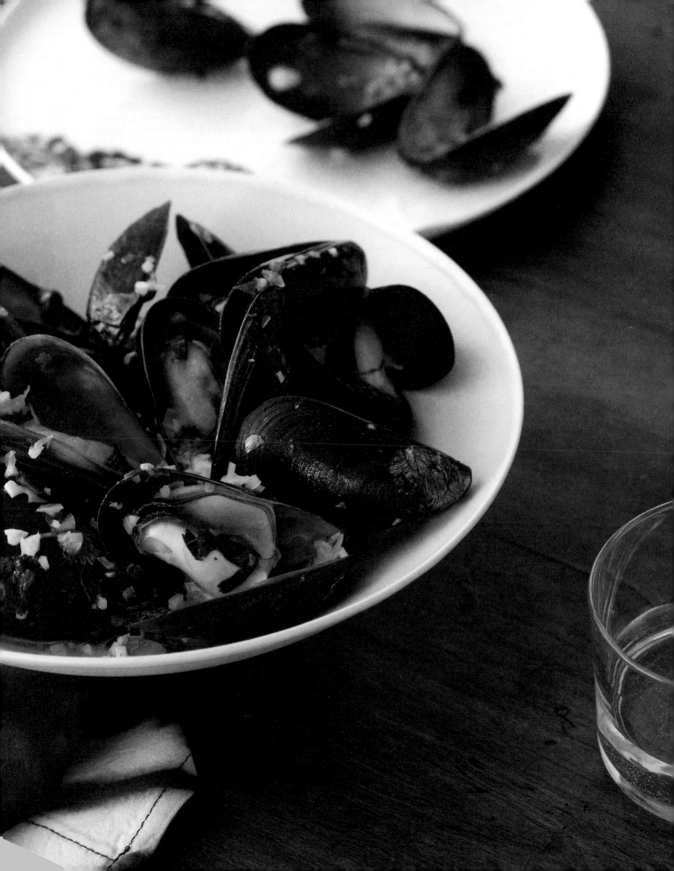

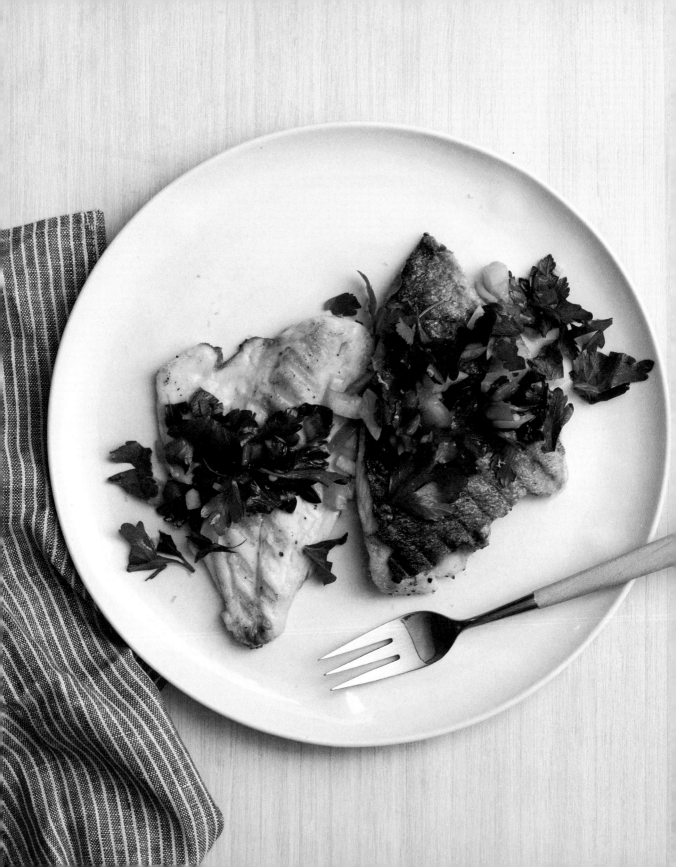

Red Mullet with Preserved Lemon and Parsley

4

Preserved lemons come originally from Morocco. Piquillo peppers are from Spain. And kalamata olives derive from Greece. Getting the picture? It's all about the Mediterranean, and that's where red mullet comes from too. In fact, it's been a delicacy of that part of the world since ancient Roman times. I've brought it up to date here.

Soak the preserved lemons in a bowl of ice-cold water for 1 hour, changing the water every 15 minutes. Transfer the soaked lemons to a cutting board and discard the seeds and flesh. Slice then finely chop the skins.

In a large bowl, whisk together the piquillo peppers, roasted garlic, olives, parsley, shallot, vinegar, ¼ cup of the oil, and the chopped preserved lemons. Set aside.

Drizzle the remaining 1 tablespoon oil over the red mullet fillets and season them generously with salt and black pepper.

Preheat an outdoor grill or a stovetop grill pan to medium-high heat. Coat the grill rack or pan with nonstick cooking spray and cook the red mullet for 3 to 4 minutes on one side. Flip the fish for just a kiss on the other side and remove from the heat.

To serve, arrange the cooked fish on a serving platter. Sprinkle the fish with the lemon zest and juice and spoon some of the preserved lemon sauce over the top.

2 preserved lemons

2 canned piquillo peppers, seeded and finely chopped

8 Roasted Garlic cloves (page 93), lightly mashed

¼ cup thinly sliced green olives

¼ cup thinly sliced kalamata olives

1 cup flat-leaf parsley leaves

1 shallot, diced

1 tablespoon red wine vinegar

¼ cup plus 1 tablespoon olive oil

4 skinless red mullet fillets (4 to 6 ounces each)

Salt and freshly ground black pepper

Grated zest and juice of 2 lemons

PER SERVING: 371 calories, 24 g protein, 16 g carbohydrates, 25 g total fat (4 g saturated), 56 mg cholesterol, 3 g fiber, 583 mg sodium

Marinated Shrimp with Scallions and Chili Water

Chili water is a Hawaiian specialty, and it gives this colorful, vibrantly flavored dish just the right addition of heat. I find the combination very comforting and Zen-like, like *feng shui* for my plate.

To make the chili water: In a blender or food processor, combine the oil, chili paste, agave nectar, salt, pepper, and 1 cup of water. Blend on a low setting until smooth and set aside.

To marinate the shrimp: In a large bowl, combine the ginger, shallots, garlic, cilantro, sesame seeds, lime zest and juice, soy sauce, and sesame oil. Add the shrimp and toss to coat in the marinade. Cover the bowl with plastic wrap and refrigerate for at least 30 minutes but no longer than 2 hours.

In a large skillet, heat the olive oil over medium-high heat. Using a slotted spoon and allowing most of the marinade to drain back into the bowl, transfer the shrimp to the pan and cook, stirring frequently, for 15 to 20 seconds. Add the scallions and cook, stirring frequently, until the shrimp are opaque, 1 to 2 minutes.

Add the chili water to the pan and cook until heated through, 1 to 2 minutes. Season to taste with salt and pepper.

PER SERVING: 382 calories, 38 g protein, 13 g carbohydrates, 21 g total fat (3 g saturated), 333 mg cholesterol, 2 g fiber, 1,031 mg sodium

CHILI WATER
- 2 tablespoons olive oil
- 1 tablespoon chili paste
- 1 tablespoon agave nectar
- 1 teaspoon fine sea salt
- ½ teaspoon freshly ground black pepper

MARINADE AND SHRIMP
- ¼ cup finely chopped fresh ginger
- 2 shallots, diced
- 4 garlic cloves, smashed and finely chopped
- ¼ cup chopped cilantro
- 2 tablespoons black sesame seeds
- Grated zest and juice of 2 limes
- ⅓ cup low-sodium soy sauce
- 3 tablespoons toasted sesame oil
- 1½ pounds large shrimp, peeled and deveined
- 2 tablespoons olive oil
- 2 bunches scallions, cut on the diagonal into ½-inch pieces
- Salt and freshly ground black pepper

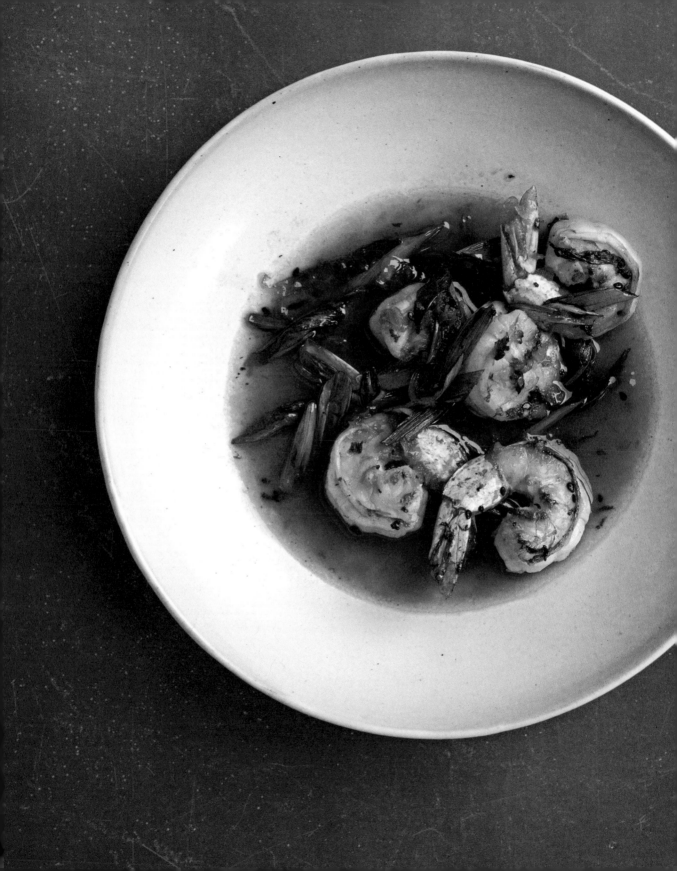

Fluke with Vietnamese Vinaigrette

 Flounder and fluke are plentiful in the summer off the shores of Montauk, and the local fisherman delivers his catch to the Surf Lodge—usually still flopping around in his cooler. If you're squeamish about baking the fish whole, use fluke fillets instead; just be sure to reduce the oven time to 4 to 6 minutes. The vinaigrette packs some intense, bright flavors that really make this dish amazing; you'll have some left over, so splash it on anything that needs a kick of flavor, from salad greens to grilled chicken.

To make the vinaigrette: In a large bowl, whisk together the vinegar, lime zest and juice, lemon zest and juice, agave nectar, soy sauce, ginger, garlic, shallot, cilantro, basil, lemongrass, chili paste, Chinese mustard, and sesame seeds. Slowly stream the oils into the rest of the ingredients, whisking constantly until well incorporated.

To cook the fish: Preheat the oven to 375°F. Line a baking sheet with parchment paper.

Place the fish on the baking sheet. Season well with salt and pepper and drizzle with the oil. Bake until the fish flakes easily with a fork, 10 to 12 minutes.

To serve, carefully scrape or lift off the skin on one side of the fish, and use a table knife to separate the fillet from the bones. Use a spatula to transfer the fillet to a plate, then lift off the tail, bones, and head from the remaining fillet. Transfer the second fillet to a plate, leaving the skin behind. Serve the fish with a couple of tablespoons of the vinaigrette drizzled on top.

PER SERVING: 336 calories, 32 g protein, 8 g carbohydrates, 20 g total fat (3 g saturated), 79 mg cholesterol, 1 g fiber, 214 mg sodium

VINAIGRETTE

¼ cup rice vinegar

Grated zest and juice of 2 limes

2 tablespoons agave nectar

1 tablespoon low-sodium soy sauce

1 teaspoon finely grated fresh ginger

2 garlic cloves, finely chopped

1 shallot, diced

2 tablespoons chopped cilantro

2 tablespoons chopped fresh basil leaves

1 tablespoon chopped lemongrass

1 tablespoon chili paste

1 teaspoon Chinese mustard

4 tablespoons black sesame seeds, toasted

½ cup extra-virgin olive oil

2 tablespoons toasted sesame oil

FLUKE

2-pound fluke, cleaned

Salt and freshly ground black pepper

2 tablespoons extra-virgin olive oil

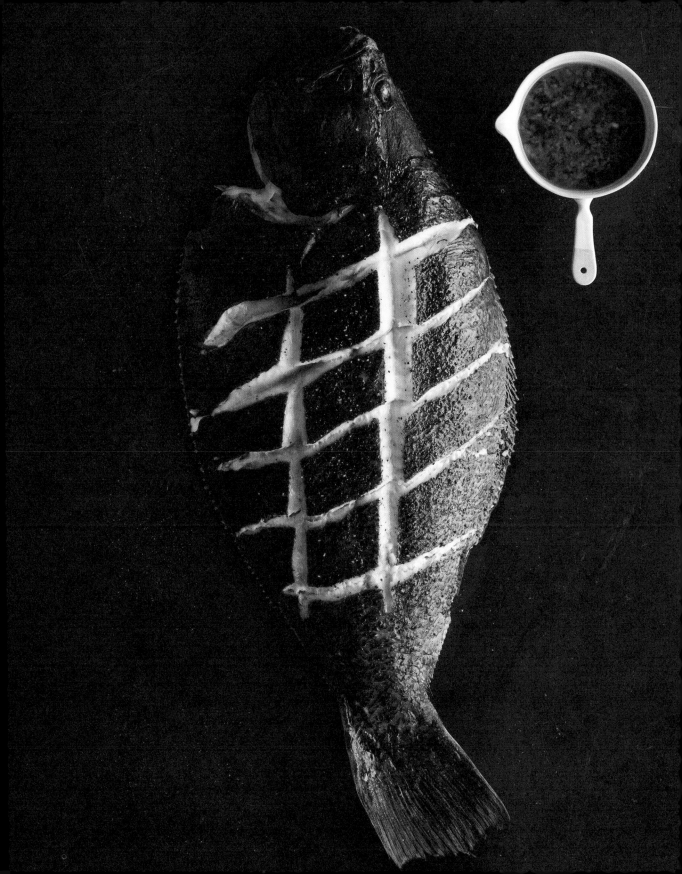

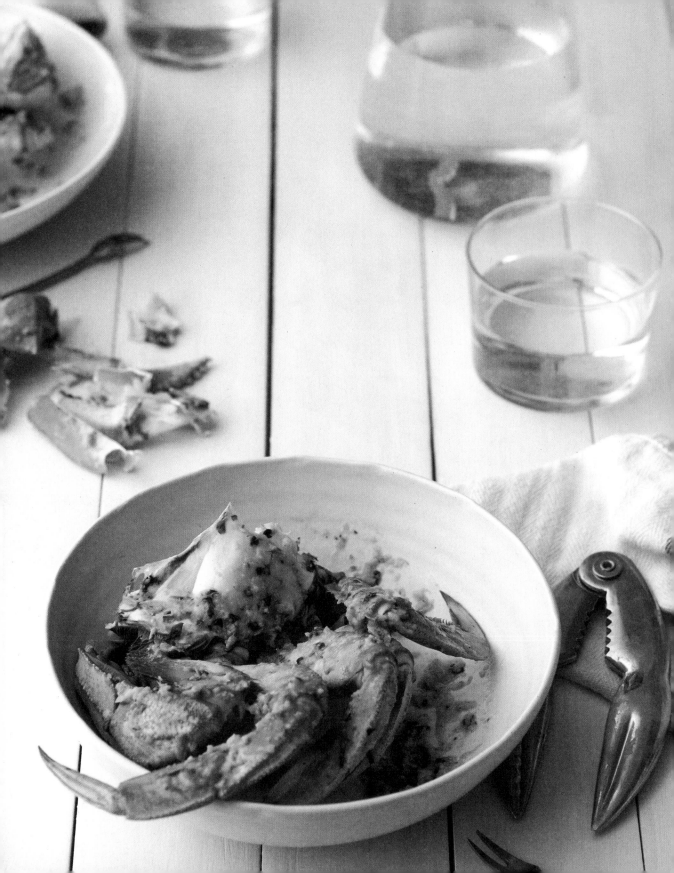

Dungeness Crab with Charred Garlic-Chili Sauce

I would eat this every day for the rest of my life if I could. Literally. (And I guess there's no reason I can't.) The charred chili sauce is so good I would serve it with steamed clams or mussels, or spread it on toasts and top with charred bok choy for some radically delicious bruschetta.

To make the garlic-chili sauce: In a blender, combine the roasted and fresh garlic with the scallions, shallot, ginger, Szechuan pepper, fish sauce, chili paste, wine, oil, and ⅓ cup water. Blend on high speed until puréed. Add the fennel and cilantro and blend for 1 minute until just incorporated but still a bit chunky. Transfer to a saucepan and set aside.

To cook the crabs: Fill a large pot two-thirds full with water. Add the lemons, bay leaves, cinnamon sticks, pepper flakes, salt, and black pepper. Bring to a boil over medium-high heat, add the live crabs and boil until the crab shells turn red, 10 to 12 minutes. Using tongs, remove the crabs from the pot and set them aside to cool. Heat the garlic-chili sauce over low heat to warm through.

When the crabs are cool enough to handle, pry off and discard the large top shells. Discard the gills and innards, then rinse the crabs under tepid running water. Set the crabs on a cutting board and cut them in half, exposing the meat.

Place a crab half on each of 4 plates and serve doused with the chili sauce.

PER SERVING: 430 calories, 18 g protein, 27 g carbohydrates, 30 g total fat (4.2 g saturated), 48 mg cholesterol, 7 g fiber, 1,021 mg sodium

CHARRED GARLIC-CHILI SAUCE

- 8 Roasted Garlic cloves (page 93), lightly mashed
- 2 garlic cloves, finely chopped
- 1 bunch scallions, thinly sliced
- 1 shallot, chopped
- 2 tablespoons grated ginger
- 1 tablespoon ground Szechuan peppercorns
- 1 teaspoon fish sauce
- 1 teaspoon sambal oelek chili paste
- ½ cup dry white wine
- ½ cup olive oil
- 1 large fennel bulb (about 1 pound), stalks discarded, cored, and finely chopped
- ¾ cup chopped fresh cilantro

CRAB

- 2 lemons, halved
- 2 bay leaves
- 2 cinnamon sticks
- 2 tablespoons red pepper flakes
- 1 teaspoon fine sea salt
- ½ teaspoon freshly ground black pepper
- 2 live Dungeness crabs

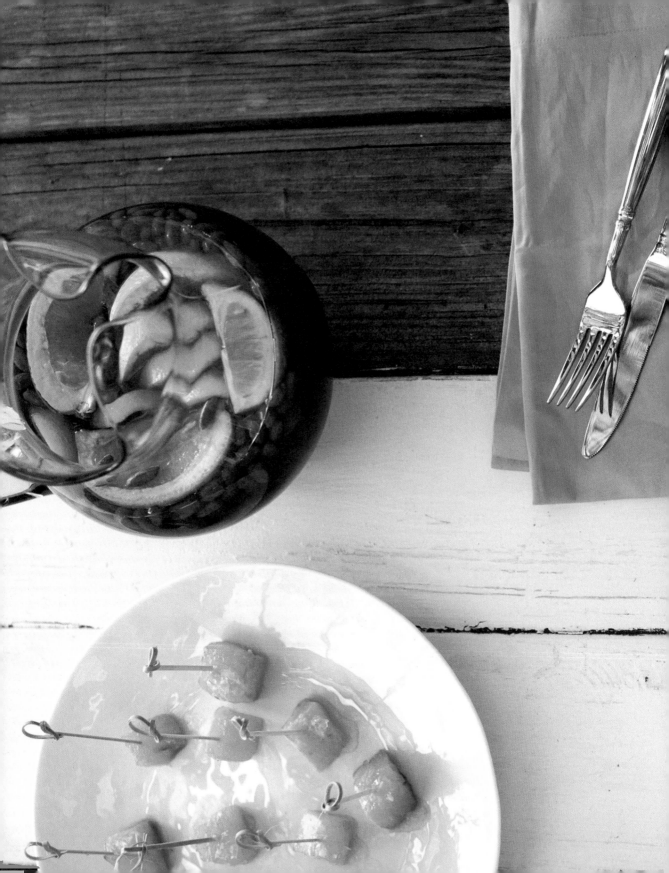

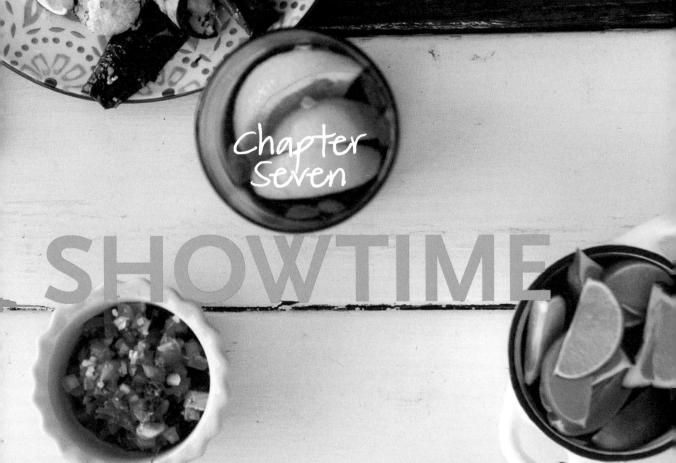

Chapter
Seven

SHOWTIME

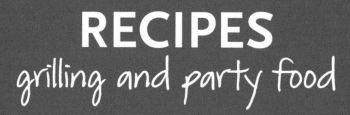

RECIPES
grilling and party food

I love the fact that casual entertaining has by and large replaced the stuffy, performance-piece dinner parties of a decade ago. Backyard barbecues, kitchen counter get-togethers—these are low-stress occasions that make everyone feel comfortable, relaxed, and part of the action, including the cook. But just because the vibe is chilled out, don't phone it in on the food front; having people into your home to share a meal is a great opportunity to go a little wild, let loose your creativity, show some flair.

Maybe because I try to spend as much of my downtime outside as I possibly can, grilling is really my entertaining mode of choice. Whether it's in Montauk with the sand and salt from a day of surfing still in my hair, or in a friend's backyard, terrace, or rooftop in the city, firing up the grill and rounding things out with some really vibrant fresh salads and veggie dishes seems to make me and my friends happiest. Add some great music, a cocktail or two (more on that in a bit), and one of the desserts from Chapter 8 and you have a recipe for a really great night.

Such occasions can of course be challenging for those of us with diabetes. "Letting yourself go" is something we cannot do—at least not often, and not too far. As fun as such indulgence may seem in the moment, ultimately it just isn't worth it. The downside is just too hard on our systems and makes us too damn sick. So in many ways, approaching a party or night out or holiday gathering is a little like walking on eggshells: We have to step very carefully. As always, it's a matter of watching our blood sugar level and taking action if it goes off the norm one way or the other.

But that doesn't mean we never party. Not at all.

BOOZE

And that brings me to the subject of alcohol. In general, I'm for it. The lunch and dinner recipes in this chapter—hell, in the whole book!—all benefit from being accompanied by the right wines. An aperitif before the meal and a brandy or marc afterward also sound great. A Bloody Mary will enliven any of the brunch dishes. So will a mimosa or bellini or even a cosmopolitan. It all sounds absolutely delicious, but if you're a diabetic, it also sounds dangerous.

Diabetics and alcohol don't mix, right? Right. And for good reason. Alcohol can cause our blood sugar to rise or, strangely enough, to drop. In fact, alcohol in excess can send blood sugar levels plummeting—sometimes dangerously. Alcohol can interfere with insulin,

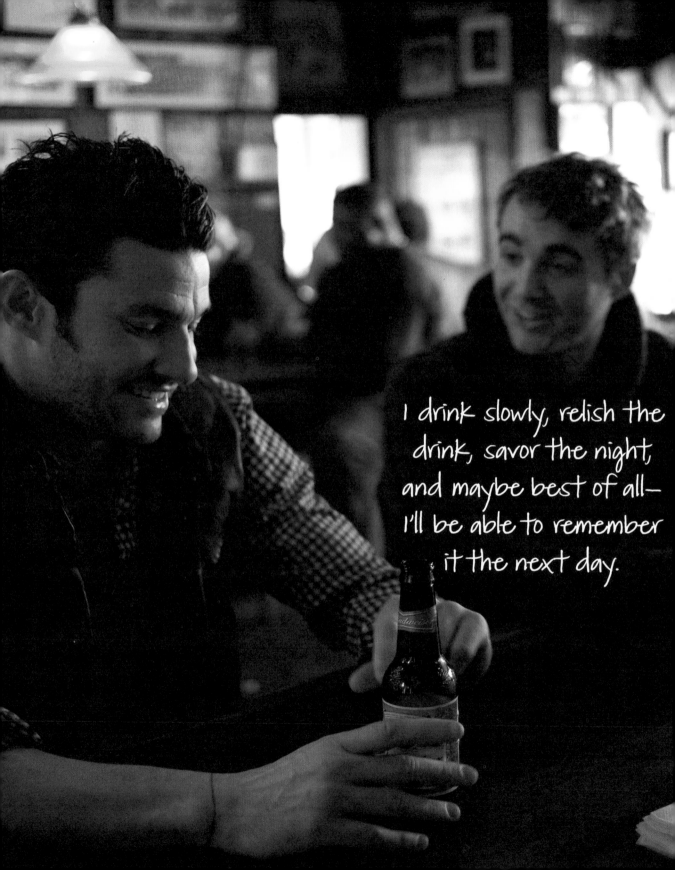

I drink slowly, relish the drink, savor the night, and maybe best of all—I'll be able to remember it the next day.

increase blood pressure, and increase triglyceride levels. It can make us feel fuzzy-brained to the point of forgetting to check our blood sugar—or just tossing the whole idea out the window. So altogether, for us, alcohol is simply not a path to health.

But the ruling principle of the Sweet Life prevails here as elsewhere—namely, everything in moderation, even alcohol. If I spend my night off with friends at the local bar, with music blaring and chilled tequila, and I drink every round offered to me over the course of a night, I will very likely end up miserably sick—if not dead. But living the Sweet Life means that there are times when I need to be with my friends, so I go to the bar on my terms, mixing in and mixing it up with a little more cushion and a little more caution than

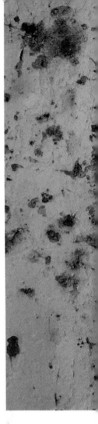

Sam's Half-Dozen Drinking Tips

1. Keep in mind that alcohol stimulates the palate and makes you hungry, so watch out for unnecessary snacking and late-night stuffing of your face.
2. Drink wine only with meals. Sip it.
3. Avoid brown alcohol, dessert wines, cordials, or juice-mixed cocktails.
4. Follow each alcoholic drink with a glass of water. This doesn't just keep you hydrated, it makes it far less likely that you'll get smashed.
5. Make it a point to check your blood sugar every other hour. This bears repeating:
6. Make it a point to check your blood sugar every other hour.

the next guy. That goes for all of us diabetics in any social setting—from a night at the pub to a black-tie blowout to a bonfire on the beach. Wherever and whatever showtime is happening, we need to be part of it because it's part of life, and being part of it means not just dealing with alcohol but accepting it.

So how do you party your head off and stay healthy and safe? Here's how I do it.

First of all, my usual obsessiveness about checking my blood sugar level kicks into even higher gear when I'm at a party.

Also, I drink selectively. I tend in general to avoid most brown liquors and have just a very occasional beer (preferably a light beer); these drinks typically have a higher sugar content than I need to deal with. Instead, I stick to vodka or gin—with club soda, not tonic or juice. Again, the aim is to keep the sugar content down.

But the key for me is staying hydrated, and my trick for that is to follow a one-to-one alcohol-to-water drinking ratio. That means one alcoholic drink—say, a vodka and soda—then sitting the next round out with a glass of water. A bit later I can do another vodka,

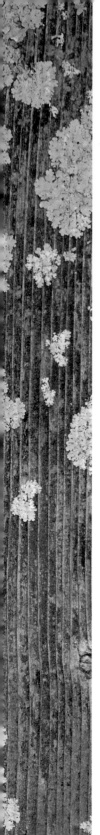

Snap It Up

Ginger is one of the key spices in a lot of my recipes. Like many people, I grew up associating it primarily with cookies out of a box. No more. Now you can find fresh ginger year-round almost everywhere, and I use it in just about anything and everything.

I'm not alone in that. Although ginger originally comes from the Far East, it has been used for centuries in Africa and the Caribbean; and in Europe it was believed to be a remedy against the Plague. Actually, it's amazingly good for you: It's an antioxidant and has anti-inflammatory properties, plus it's a source of potassium, magnesium, copper, manganese, and vitamin B_6. And as anyone who has ever been seasick knows, it's about the only thing that will do any good at all against motion sickness—and against other kinds of nausea too.

But it's the taste of it I love—pungent, spicy, and suffused with that very specific aroma. The cookie is not wrongly named: Ginger brings a certain sudden snap—a real pizzazz—to any food it's part of. I use it regularly to spice vegetable and fish dishes and in a very festive meat dish you'll find on page 207. It's a spice that can really enliven a dish, so I urge you to be creative with it; it's a great way to play with your food.

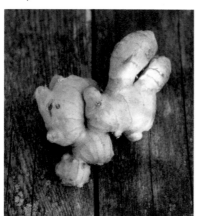

followed by another glass of water. This way I'm staying hydrated and I'm also avoiding getting totally plastered. I know from unhappy experience that if I don't stick to this alternating booze-water pattern, the next day will be dramatic. By "dramatic" I mean propped over the toilet tossing my guts up and swearing I'll never drink again. Trust me.

Meanwhile, I'm checking my blood level. I'm also having a good time. I'm enjoying myself. I drink slowly, relish the drink, savor the night, and maybe best of all—I'll be able to remember it the next day.

On a recent Saturday night I got to a party at a little after 11:00, having had a light, low-carb snack—usually it's something vegetable-based, like some sautéed greens to keep my blood sugar on an even keel—at about 10:30, after things had calmed down in the restaurant. I had my first vodka and soda when I arrived at the party, then a long glass of water, and at midnight, I checked my blood sugar. All clear. So I sipped another vodka. By the time I left a little past 3:30 a.m., I had had three vodka and sodas and at least five glasses of water, and I had checked my blood sugar three times. That's about average—standard operating procedure for me at a party, and a standard amount of alcohol imbibed. And for me it was a win-win. I had a hell of a night, I felt great, and there was no hangover in the morning. Sweet.

EAT HEALTHY TO STAY HEALTHY

Staying healthy at a party, during the holiday season, or on any festive occasion is good for everyone. Too much sugar in the blood is bad for everybody, not just for us diabetics. Too much rich food makes a lot of people feel sleepy, and too much food altogether—too much eating!—makes everybody feel bloated. The traditional loosening of the belt after Thanksgiving dinner, accompanied in many families by the loud vow to never eat another morsel, may be an inherent part of the holiday, but even once a year it's not particularly good for us. And let's face it: It's never just once a year.

The recipes in this chapter all make healthy meals. They're low-calorie, low-carb, offering healthy protein in good proportion to vegetables and fruit.

Let yourself go a bit when you prepare these dishes. You should enjoy making these foods as much as you—and your guests—enjoy eating them. That's what festive times are all about.

The World of Ceviche

How varied—and how open to creativity—is the world of cooking? For openers, just consider the world of ceviche. Regarded as virtually the "national dish" of Peru, raw fish marinated in a citrus-based mixture is popular through much of South America and also appears in various forms around the Pacific, including virtually all the island nations of the Pacific, and the Caribbean as well. Here are just a few of the best-known variations (see page 193 for my Crab Ceviche recipe, too.)

Peru: Typically made with bass, Peruvian ceviche is usually marinated for several hours in a mixture of Key lime or orange juice with onions, chiles, and other seasonings to taste. A contemporary variant uses the same ingredients but the fish is marinated for just a few minutes, more like a Japanese sashimi.

Ecuador: Here shrimp ceviche is the rule, and the marinade includes tomato sauce.

Chile: Grapefruit juice is often used in the marinade, along with garlic, mint, and cilantro.

Guatemala: They love clams in Guatemala, and throw just about anything, including very picante sauce, into the marinade.

Mexico: Add avocado and cilantro to the marinade then wrap a few spoonfuls in a tortilla for a Mexican twist.

The Bahamas: Here they add bell pepper lightly cooked shellfish to make conch salad, the Caribbean version of this ubiquitous dish.

The Philippines: Filipino chefs marinate the raw fish in vinegar and add garlic, onions, ginger, and lots of spices.

Pan-Pacific: Across the Pacific, raw fish is marinated in—why not?—coconut milk, along with citrus, onions, and spices. It's often served in the coconut shell.

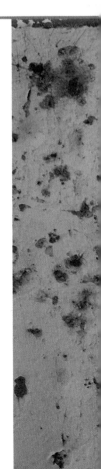

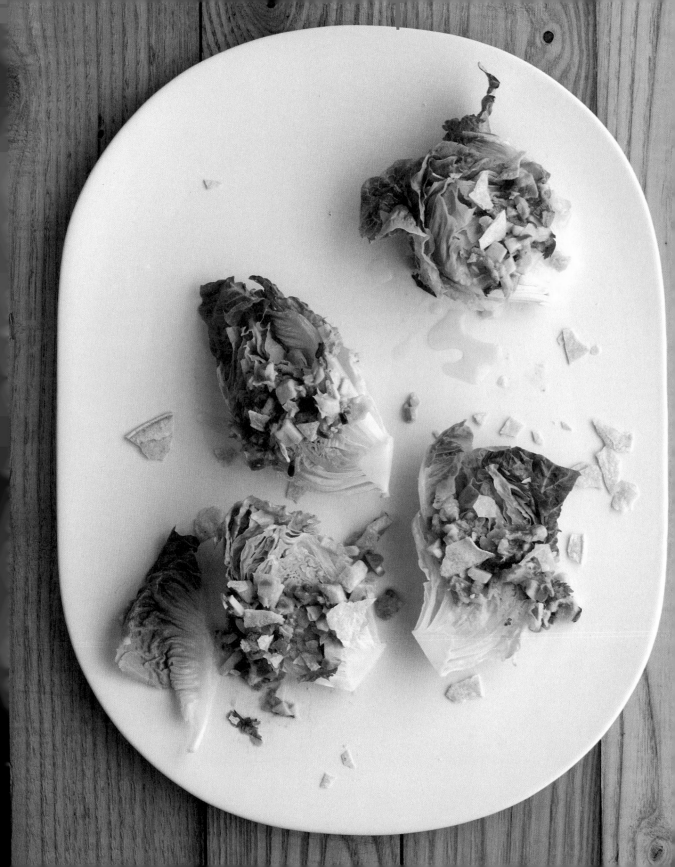

Lettuce wedge Salad with Avocado-Tortilla Vinaigrette

 4

Boston or Bibb lettuce offers a crunch like no other, and I love it when the lettuce still has a few ice-cold drops of water that burst in your mouth on that first bite. Offer this up as a first course or even as a second alongside a grilled protein like skirt steak or chicken. Regular iceberg lettuce works as well; just cut the whole head into quarters. Make the vinaigrette right before you serve the salads so the tortillas don't lose their crunch and the avocado stays green.

In a large skillet, heat the garlic oil over medium-high heat. Add the onion, garlic, and coriander seeds and cook, stirring frequently, until the onion is translucent, 2 to 3 minutes. Add the jalapeño and cook for about 30 more seconds. Set aside to cool to room temperature.

Once the vegetables have cooled, transfer to a medium bowl and stir in the yogurt, lime zest and juice, vinegar, and cilantro, whisking constantly until well combined. Crumble the tortilla chips into the vinaigrette mixture. Halve, pit, peel, and dice the avocados and add them in, tossing to combine.

Halve (or quarter) the heads of lettuce and arrange on salad plates. Spoon the vinaigrette over the wedges and serve immediately.

PER SERVING: 220 calories, 3 g protein, 12 g carbohydrates, 20 g total fat (3 g saturated), 0 mg cholesterol, 5 g fiber, 28 mg sodium

¼ cup Roasted Garlic Oil (page 93)

½ large red onion, finely diced

2 garlic cloves, smashed and finely chopped

1½ teaspoons coriander seeds

1 tablespoon seeded and finely diced jalapeño pepper or to taste

2 teaspoons low-fat plain yogurt

Grated zest and juice of 1 lime

1½ tablespoons red wine vinegar

¼ cup chopped fresh cilantro

8 white corn tortilla chips

1 Hass avocado

2 heads Boston or Bibb lettuce or 1 head iceberg lettuce, rinsed and chilled

Guacamole with Feta Cheese and Almonds

We all love guac any time of the day or night, rain or shine, snow or waves, right? I do! But I wanted to give it a fresh spin, a new face—call it a makeover! After countless efforts mixing this with that and that with this, here is, by far, the winner. It's got flavor and punch and is the type of snack that is good anytime, anywhere. Put some in a baggie on ice and take it on a road trip with some blue corn chips, and you will never again be tempted by those fast-food and gas-station junk food emporiums. Note: This isn't supposed to be a smooth guacamole—the tomatoes should stay chunky. Also, avocados are definitely necessary for a balanced diet—thank goodness!

In a food processor, process the almonds until coarsely ground.

Halve the avocados, pit, and scoop the flesh into a medium bowl. Add the lemon zest and juice, hot sauce, onion, feta, and ground almonds. Mix until well combined, mashing the avocado with the back of a spoon. Fold in the tomatoes and oil. Transfer to a serving dish and season to taste with salt and pepper.

PER SERVING: 210 calories, 4 g protein, 12 g carbohydrates, 18 g total fat (3 g saturated), 5 mg cholesterol, 6 g fiber, 85 mg sodium

½ cup sliced almonds, toasted in the oven

4 Hass avocados

Grated zest and juice of 3 lemons

6 to 8 dashes of hot sauce

1 small red onion, diced

⅓ cup feta cheese

2 medium vine-ripened tomatoes, seeded and diced

2 tablespoons Roasted Garlic Oil (page 93)

Salt and freshly ground black pepper

Grilled Vegetables with Ricotta Salata, Olive Oil, and Lemon

 I think vegetable crudités are great, but as a chef you can't just serve a bunch of raw carrots and broccoli to someone and say "Bon app," you know? These vegetables have been dolled up a bit with everyday items. Your guests will definitely appreciate these a lot more than the typical spread of veggie dippers with ranch dressing!

In a large bowl, combine the zucchini, peppers, onion, broccoli, cauliflower, parsley, and basil. Add the vinegar and garlic oil and toss gently to coat. Cover the bowl with plastic wrap and marinate the vegetables in the refrigerator for at least 30 minutes.

Preheat an outdoor grill or a stovetop grill pan to medium-high heat.

Grill the vegetables in batches until they are all charred on both sides, 4 to 6 minutes total per batch. Remove the vegetables from the grill, transfer them to a serving platter, and chill in the refrigerator for 1 hour.

To serve, remove the vegetables from the refrigerator. Season to taste with salt and black pepper. Grate the cheese over the vegetables, drizzle with the extra-virgin olive oil, and sprinkle with the lemon juice.

PER SERVING: 139 calories, 4 g protein, 10 g carbohydrates, 10 g total fat (2 g saturated), 6 mg cholesterol, 3 g fiber, 146 mg sodium

- **2 large zucchini, each cut lengthwise into 8 slices**
- **2 red bell peppers, cut lengthwise into 8 slices**
- **1 large red onion, cut crosswise into ¼-inch-thick rings**
- **2 cups broccoli florets**
- **2 cups cauliflower florets**
- **½ cup chopped flat-leaf parsley**
- **½ cup chopped fresh basil**
- **¼ cup red wine vinegar**
- **½ cup Roasted Garlic Oil (page 93)**
- **Salt and freshly ground black pepper**
- **2 ounces ricotta salata cheese**
- **1 tablespoon good quality extra-virgin olive oil**
- **Juice of 1 lemon**

Tuna Ceviche with Grapefruit and Mustard

 4

This is similar to a traditional ceviche, but it is fast and pretty—like tuna itself—the way we like it. It just says "summer" with every bite, but don't get too laid back: The mustard gives it a kick as well.

In a large bowl, combine the chives, grapefruit, orange juice, mustard oil, Dijon mustard, and honey. Add the tuna and toss gently to combine, making sure the tuna is well coated and the grapefruit segments stay whole. Season to taste with salt and pepper.

PER SERVING: 132 calories, 14 g protein, 10 g carbohydrates, 4 g total fat (0.5 g saturated), 25 mg cholesterol, 1 g fiber, 52 mg sodium

- 8 **fresh chives, finely chopped**
- 1 **red or white grapefruit, peeled and segmented**

   Juice of 1 orange
- 1 **tablespoon mustard oil**
- 1 **teaspoon Dijon mustard**
- 1 **teaspoon orange blossom honey**
- 8 **ounces fresh tuna, cut into ½-inch cubes**

   Salt and freshly ground black pepper

Crab Ceviche with Blueberries and Popcorn

 Crab may be my favorite food of all time—except maybe for scallops or octopus—and I like it any way I can get it, including in this totally kicky ceviche dish. I know this combination of foods sounds totally off the wall, but I love to play with food, and this play knocks it out of the park. Trust me! (And if you don't want to trust me, trust the diners at The Surf Lodge, where this dish is a top seller and the one people always ask for.)

In a medium bowl, whisk together the salt, pepper, ginger, garlic, cinnamon, cumin, agave nectar, yuzu juice, lemon zest and juice, and the oil. Using a rubber spatula, carefully fold in the crab and blueberries.

To serve, spoon the ceviche into bowls and garnish with a handful of popcorn per serving.

PER SERVING: 229 calories, 19 g protein, 20 g carbohydrates, 8 g total fat (1 g saturated), 80 mg cholesterol, 4 g fiber, 344 mg sodium

1 teaspoon fine sea salt

½ teaspoon freshly ground black pepper

2 tablespoons finely chopped fresh ginger

1 tablespoon finely chopped garlic

2 tablespoons ground cinnamon

2 tablespoons ground cumin

2 tablespoons agave nectar

¾ cup yuzu juice

Grated zest and juice of 4 lemons

3 tablespoons olive oil

1 pound fresh jumbo lump crabmeat

1 pint blueberries

1 cup plain popcorn

The Fish Fry

This dish is the foundation of all things Southern. All things Low Country. Hell—all things American! Is this the poster child for health eating? No, but it is fun every once in awhile. Not three times-a-week fun or even three times a month. It's the kind of fun that happens once or twice a summer or on a really chilly evening in the winter. Remember, even diabetics can party—as with everything else, in moderation. Sweet.

Back home they serve breaded or battered fried fish with coleslaw or hush puppies and sweet iced tea. Way sweet. I've seen people pour a pitcher of sugar into the tea. I leave that stuff out and focus on the necessary. So here's a cleaned-up recipe so we can enjoy American-style fish fry minus the sweet tea and super-fried fish. Flash frying helps reduce the fat content, and fresh lemon at the end is key. The fresh juice supplies the extra boost that makes the whole thing work. You can use any mild white fish that is readily accessible. Don't get hung up on what kind of fish; the question really should be how fresh it is.

In a shallow bowl, whisk together the buttermilk, eggs, paprika, garlic powder, onion powder, Old Bay seasoning, ½ teaspoon salt, ¼ teaspoon pepper, and hot sauce. Add the cornmeal to another shallow bowl.

Dip each fish fillet into the buttermilk mixture and then the cornmeal to coat on both sides. Shake off any excess cornmeal.

In a large skillet, heat the oil over medium-high heat. Add the fillets and cook until they are golden brown and flake easily with a fork, about 3 minutes per side. Sprinkle the fish with the lemon zest and juice and season to taste with salt and pepper. Serve hot.

PER SERVING: 385 calories, 47 g protein, 26 g carbohydrates, 10 g total fat (2 g saturated), 166 mg cholesterol, 1 g fiber, 393 mg sodium

- 2 cups buttermilk
- 3 cage-free organic eggs, lightly beaten
- 1 tablespoon paprika
- 1 tablespoon garlic powder
- 1 tablespoon onion
- 1 tablespoon Old Bay seasoning
- Salt and freshly ground black pepper
- 1 tablespoon hot sauce
- 2 cups cornmeal
- 12 tilapia fillets (about 8 ounces each)
- 1 cup canola oil
- Grated zest and juice of 2 lemons

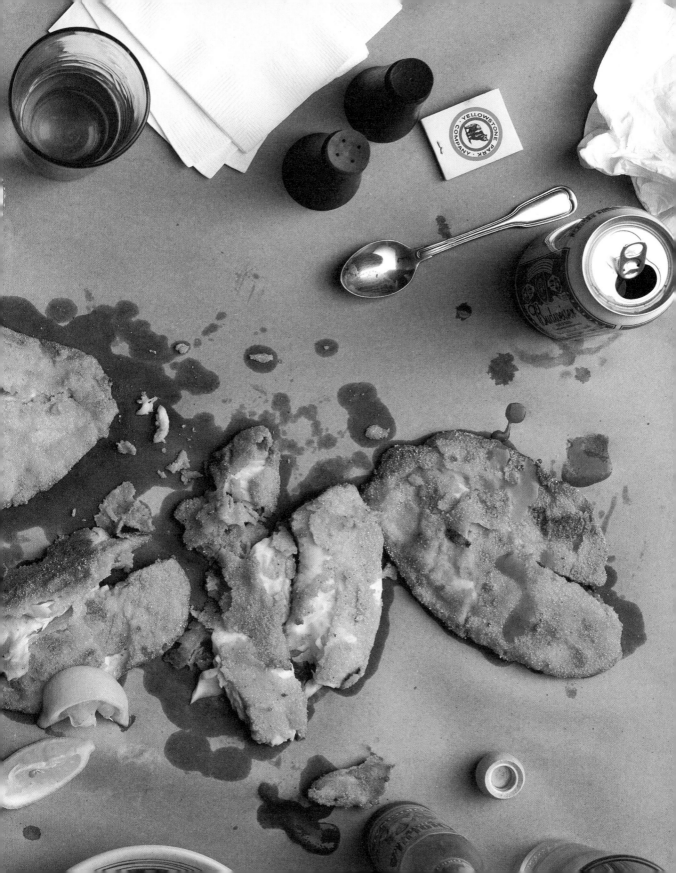

Oyster Roast

(4)

Oyster roasts in Charleston, South Carolina, are epic. Live music, people everywhere, ice-cold beer, and local oysters. Among the festivities are shucking competitions and eating contests, but the best part is getting the huge buckets of steamed oysters with crackers, hot sauce, and lemon and just hanging out on a picnic blanket eating them. When I'm in New York, I like to think about the palms, the pluff mud, as we call our dark marsh soil, and that salty seaweed smell in the morning. But you don't have to be in Charleston to make this recipe. Just make sure you're with a great group of friends, that you've got some special spirits, and that you're in the mood for fun! You can sub in clams or mussels if you like—just keep in mind that the mussels cook much faster.

In a large soup pot or Dutch oven, heat the garlic oil over medium heat. Add the garlic, celery, onion, sweet potato, and fennel and cook, stirring frequently, until the potatoes and fennel are fork-tender, 3 to 4 minutes.

Increase the heat to high. Add the wine and cook for 2 minutes, scraping up any browned bits from the bottom of the pan to deglaze it. Add the milk, Worcestershire sauce, and hot sauce and bring to a simmer. Add the corn and cook for 5 minutes. Add the parsley and oysters, cover the pot, and steam until the corn is tender and the oysters are nice and plump and semi-firm to the touch, about 4 minutes.

Ladle the oysters and vegetables into 4 large soup bowls, with one corn half per serving, and season to taste with salt and pepper.

PER SERVING: 512 calories, 33 g protein, 53 g carbohydrates, 18 g total fat (3 g saturated), 150 mg cholesterol, 8 g fiber, 661 mg sodium

3 tablespoons Roasted Garlic Oil (page 93)

8 garlic cloves, smashed and finely chopped

8 celery ribs, cut on the diagonal into ½-inch-thick slices

1 large onion, finely sliced

1 sweet potato, peeled and cubed

1 large fennel bulb (about 1 pound), stalks discarded, cored, and thinly sliced

½ cup dry white wine

1 cup almond milk

2 tablespoons Worcestershire sauce

1 teaspoon hot sauce

2 small ears corn, husked and halved

1 cup loosely packed hand-torn flat-leaf parsley

2 dozen oysters, shucked, with their liquid

Salt and freshly ground black pepper

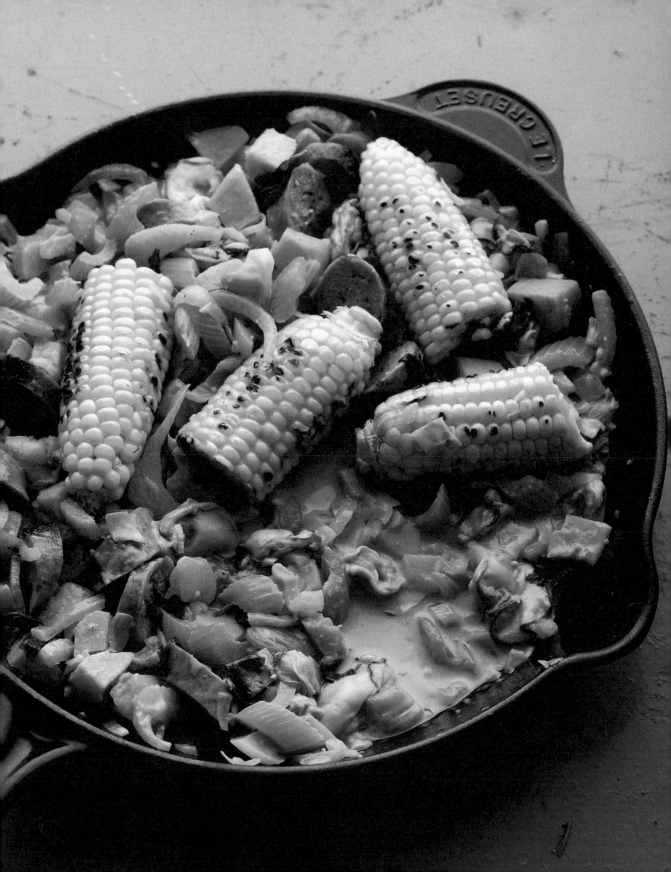

Fish Tacos with Tomato Salsa and Citrus Crema

If you haven't tried fish tacos yet, you're missing out on one of the finer things in life. I spent 2 years concocting, tweaking, throwing out, and eating thousands of these damn things until I got it right. Actually, forget "right"—until I had it bulletproof. By "bulletproof" I mean if they weren't perfect, I would have been hazed, stoned, and exiled from where I reside. At the end of the day I realized you just need three ingredients: the fish itself, the tortilla, and, just as important, the freshly shaved green cabbage; this last provides just the right amount of texture and crunch in each bite. The salsa and citrus crema bring everything together. If you don't have time to make your own fresh salsa, a good quality jarred one will do. On the West Coast, mahi-mahi is most often used to fill fish tacos, but any mild white fish, such as cod or tilapia, will work brilliantly.

Preheat the oven to 350°F. Place the butter and ¼ cup oil on a rimmed baking sheet and place it in the oven to melt the butter. When the butter is melted, arrange the fish fillets on the baking sheet and sprinkle with the parsley, cilantro, and garlic. Pour the wine around the fillets and season generously with salt and pepper.

Bake the fish until it flakes easily with a fork, 10 to 12 minutes. Break the fish into 1-inch chunks and set aside.

Heat a grill pan over high heat. Place the tortillas in the pan, one at a time, and cook until they are hot and marked with grill lines, 15 to 30 seconds. Brush the hot tortillas with a little oil and sprinkle with a little salt and pepper.

To assemble the tacos, spoon 2 tablespoons of salsa, a few fish chunks, and some of the cabbage onto each tortilla. Drizzle 1 tablespoon of the crema over each serving and top with 2 or 3 avocado slices. Season to taste with salt and pepper and serve with a lime wedge.

PER SERVING: 447 calories, 28 g protein, 42 g carbohydrates, 19 g total fat (5 g saturated), 52 mg cholesterol, 6 g fiber, 489 mg sodium

- 2 tablespoons unsalted butter, cut into small pieces
- ¼ cup olive oil, plus more for brushing the tortillas
- 2 pounds skinless cod, snapper, or mahi-mahi fillets
- ½ cup loosely packed chopped flat-leaf parsley
- ½ cup chopped fresh cilantro
- 4 garlic cloves, chopped
- ¼ cup dry white wine
- Salt and freshly ground black pepper
- 16 flour tortillas (6 inch)
- 1 cup Tomato Salsa (page 200)
- ½ large head green cabbage, thinly sliced
- ½ cup Citrus Crema (page 200)
- 1 Hass avocado, pitted, peeled, and thinly sliced
- 2 limes, cut into 4 wedges each

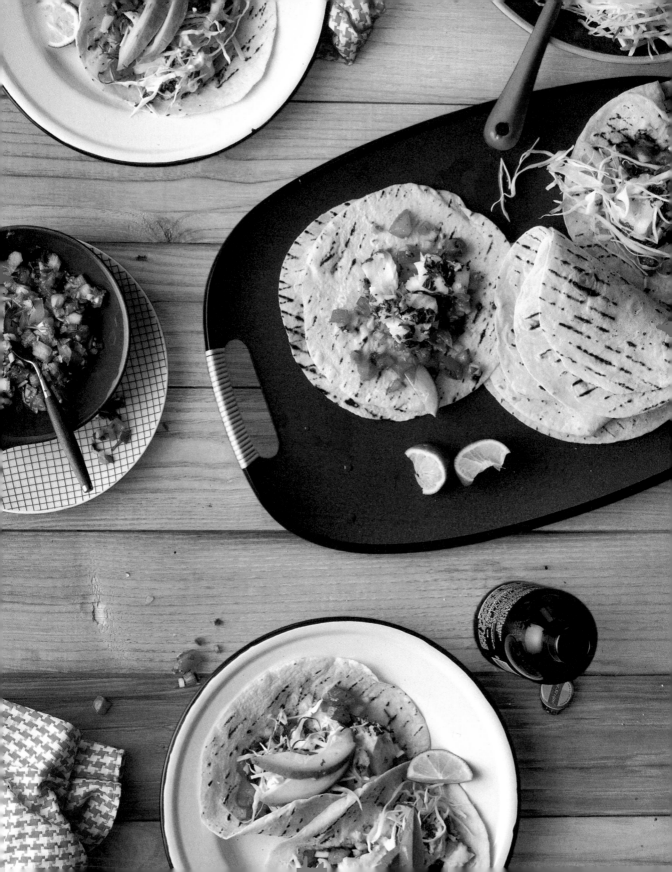

TOMATO SALSA 🍴 MAKES 2 CUPS

Place a small skillet over high heat. When it begins to smoke, add the cumin and coriander seeds and toast, stirring constantly to prevent them from burning, until fragrant, about 1 minute. Allow the seeds to cool, then use a mortar and pestle to crush them coarsely.

In a medium bowl, toss together the tomatoes, onion, cilantro, jalapeño, and lime juice. Add the crushed cumin and coriander seeds and mix well, then season to taste with salt and black pepper. The salsa can be refrigerated, covered, for up to 24 hours.

1 tablespoon cumin seeds

1 tablespoon coriander seeds

3 medium vine-ripened tomatoes, diced

1 small red onion, diced

3 tablespoons chopped fresh cilantro

½ jalapeño chile pepper, seeded and finely chopped

¼ cup fresh lime juice

Salt and freshly ground black pepper

CITRUS CREMA 🍴 MAKES 1¼ CUPS

1 lemon

1 lime

1 orange

½ cup 2% plain organic Greek yogurt

⅓ cup sour cream

Salt and freshly ground black pepper

Use a Microplane zester to zest the lemon, lime, and about half of the orange. Place the zests in a small bowl and stir in the yogurt and sour cream.

Juice all of the fruits into another small bowl. Measure out ¼ cup of their combined juice (save the rest for another use) and add to the yogurt–sour cream mixture. Stir to combine and season to taste with salt and pepper. The crema can be refrigerated, covered, for up to 2 days.

Grilled Scallops with Chimichurri

This dish is luxurious enough for a black-tie dinner and laid-back enough for a Sunday morning, and it's jam-packed with nutrients. Three florets of cauliflower a day will provide you with 67 percent of your daily vitamin C requirement. And scallops? Don't even get me started. If I had to choose only one protein to eat each day for the rest of my life, scallops would be a top contender. They're a very good source of vitamin B12, which promotes cardiovascular health, and they have rich quantities of potassium, selenium, and magnesium.

To make the chimichurri: In a medium bowl, combine the oil, vinegar, sambal, agave nectar, lemon zest and juice, salt, and pepper. Whisk well until blended. Stir in the parsley, basil, oregano, and mint. Set aside at room temperature.

To marinate the scallops: In a large bowl, whisk together the oil, turmeric, cinnamon, and Old Bay seasoning. Add the scallops, mixing well to coat in the marinade. Cover the bowl with plastic wrap and refrigerate for at least 30 minutes.

Preheat an outdoor grill or a stovetop grill pan to medium-high heat. Remove the scallops from the marinade and season them generously on both sides with salt and pepper. Grill the scallops until they are golden brown on both sides and firm to the touch, 2 minutes per side.

To serve, arrange the scallops on a serving platter and spoon about ½ cup of the chimichurri on top.

PER SERVING: 252 calories, 9 g protein, 9 g carbohydrates, 21 g total fat (3 g saturated), 15 mg cholesterol, 2 g fiber, 555 mg sodium

CHIMICHURRI

- ¼ cup olive oil
- 1 tablespoon red wine vinegar
- 1 teaspoon sambal oelek chili paste
- 1 teaspoon agave nectar
- Grated zest and juice of 2 lemons
- ½ teaspoon fine sea salt
- ¼ teaspoon freshly ground black pepper
- ½ cup loosely packed finely chopped flat-leaf parsley
- ½ cup loosely packed finely chopped fresh basil leaves
- ¼ cup finely chopped fresh oregano leaves
- ¼ cup finely chopped fresh mint leaves

SCALLOPS

- 2 tablespoons olive oil
- 1 teaspoon turmeric
- 1 teaspoon ground cinnamon
- 1 teaspoon Old Bay seasoning
- 1 dozen large sea scallops, preferably diver scallops
- Salt and freshly ground black pepper

Beef Tacos with Charred Tomatillo–Pepper Relish

6

I love a good spicy taco. The kind where a cold Corona is a must. Pepperoncini lend some good heat and a slightly pickled taste to the beef. Make these in batches for a football game or tailgating barbecue, but make enough. They're really good. Sometimes I'll put a splash of sriracha on top for even more heat; it is so good that way. If you're not worried about upping the fat content a bit, sour cream can help cool down your mouth.

TOMATILLO-PEPPER RELISH

- ½ cup diced canned tomatillos
- 4 jarred pepperoncini peppers, drained, seeded, and thinly sliced
- 2 fresh jalapeño chile peppers, seeded and thinly sliced
- Juice of 1 lime
- ½ teaspoon fine sea salt
- ¼ teaspoon freshly ground black pepper

BEEF

- 2 tablespoons canola oil
- 1 small Vidalia or other sweet onion, finely diced
- 3 celery ribs, diced
- 6 garlic cloves, smashed and finely chopped
- 1 tablespoon ground cumin
- 1 tablespoon garlic powder
- 1 tablespoon onion powder
- 1½ teaspoons Old Bay seasoning
- 1½ teaspoons chili powder
- 1½ teaspoons turmeric
- 1 pound lean ground beef
- 2 tablespoons canned crushed San Marzano tomatoes
- Salt and freshly ground black pepper

TACOS

- 6 corn tortillas (6 inch)
- 1 cup shredded iceberg lettuce
- ½ cup diced vine-ripened tomatoes
- ⅓ cup hand-torn fresh cilantro
- Salt and freshly ground black pepper
- 2 limes, cut into wedges
- Sour cream (optional)

Preheat the oven to 450°F.

To make the relish: In a small bowl, mix together the tomatillos, pepperoncini, and jalapeños. Spread the mixture evenly on a baking sheet. Bake until the tomatillos and peppers are charred, about 10 minutes. Set aside to cool.

Once the tomatillo-pepper mixture has cooled to room temperature, season it with the lime juice, salt, and pepper. Cut up the seasoned peppers to make a relish.

To prepare the beef: In a large skillet, heat the oil over medium-high heat. Add the onion, celery, chopped garlic, cumin, garlic powder, onion powder, Old Bay seasoning, chili powder, and turmeric. Cook until the onions and celery are translucent, 2 to 3 minutes.

Add the beef to the pan, reduce the heat to medium, and cook, breaking apart the meat as it cooks with a wooden spoon, until the beef is browned, 2 to 3 minutes. Add the canned crushed tomatoes and cook, stirring constantly, for 1 to 2 minutes to melt the flavors. Remove from the heat and drain off any excess grease. Season to taste with salt and pepper and set it aside.

To assemble the tacos: Heat a large skillet over medium heat and warm the tortillas one at a time for 1 to 2 minutes. Spoon some of the meat mixture into the center of each tortilla, followed by a handful of lettuce and a spoonful of the charred tomatillo-pepper relish. Top that off with the chopped fresh tomatoes, cilantro, and a dash of salt and pepper. Squeeze a lime wedge over each taco, and don't forget to reward yourself with a dollop of sour cream if you've been on the treadmill today.

PER SERVING: 310 calories, 21 g protein, 32 g carbohydrates, 11 g total fat
(2 g saturated), 147 mg cholesterol, 6 g fiber, 678 mg sodium

Grilled Chicken Thighs with Endive and Apple Sauté

 I really get annoyed when people ask for all white meat when they order chicken. It is so lame. Dark meat is better tasting, is much more flavorful, and retains more moisture throughout the cooking process. I love chicken thighs cooked on the grill with some crisp skin!! If you haven't tried them, you have no idea what you're missing. The special twist here is combining the sweetness of the apple and the classically bitter taste of the endive.

To prepare the chicken: In a large bowl, combine the vinegar, lemon juice, club soda, apple juice, soy sauce, pepper flakes, cilantro, and garlic. Add the chicken, tossing to coat well in the marinade, then cover the bowl tightly with plastic wrap and refrigerate for at least 1 hour.

Preheat the oven to 350°F.

Remove the chicken from the marinade and season generously with salt and black pepper. Place the chicken on a baking sheet and bake until golden brown, 12 to 15 minutes. Remove the chicken from the oven. In a large skillet, heat the butter over medium-high heat. Add the chicken and cook until the thighs are golden brown on both sides and a meat thermometer inserted in the thickest portion of a thigh registers 160°F, 1 to 2 minutes per side.

To cook the endive and apple: In a large skillet, heat the garlic oil over medium-high heat. When the oil begins to shimmer, add the onion, ginger, and garlic and cook, stirring frequently, until the onion is translucent, 2 to 3 minutes. Add the agave nectar, vinegar, and lemon juice and cook for 1 minute to incorporate. Add the endive, apple, and cilantro and cook until the apple is fork-tender, about 3 minutes.

Serve the chicken on top of the endives and apples and enjoy.

PER SERVING: 330 calories, 29 g protein, 22 g carbohydrates, 15 g total fat (4 g saturated), 122 mg cholesterol, 3 g fiber, 315 mg sodium

CHICKEN

- 3 tablespoons rice vinegar
- Juice of 1 lemon
- ¼ cup club soda
- ¼ cup apple juice
- ¼ cup low-sodium soy sauce
- 1 teaspoon red pepper flakes
- 1 cup chopped fresh cilantro
- 2 garlic cloves
- 8 small boneless, skinless organic chicken thighs
- Salt and freshly ground black pepper
- 1 tablespoon unsalted butter

ENDIVE AND APPLE SAUTÉ

- 2 tablespoons Roasted Garlic Oil (page 93)
- 1 red onion, thinly sliced
- 1 tablespoon grated ginger
- 1 tablespoon chopped garlic
- 2 tablespoons agave nectar
- 2 tablespoons rice vinegar
- Juice of 1 lemon
- 2 cups chopped Belgian endive
- 1 apple, peeled and diced
- ¼ cup chopped fresh cilantro

Lemon Chicken with Lemongrass and Love

 6

This lemon chicken comes to you courtesy of Brittney, one of the lovely bundles of joy in the kitchen at The Surf Lodge. It would be a huge hit for a family picnic or to bring to a potluck dinner or other cool gathering. It knocks the daylights out of any other lemon chicken you've ever had. It's so refreshing and so damn simple. And we all know about lemongrass—how it's a cancer-fighting grass as well as a key herb in Asian cuisines. I have a kind of obsession with lemongrass. I admit it's almost creepy. Like if lemongrass had a phone, I'd totally text her and be like, so, what-ya-doin'-later kind of obsession. But it's the best. Not only is its flavor a necessary addition to so many dishes—it's all over Vietnamese and Thai cooking—but it perfumes anything it touches with unique hints of lemon and ginger. It is intense and I love it.

In a large bowl combine the lemon zest and slices, lemon juice, orange zest, oil, vinegar, basil, parsley, garlic, ginger, lemongrass, and lemon-pepper seasoning. Add the chicken, turning to coat well in the marinade, then cover the bowl tightly with plastic wrap and refrigerate for at least 4 and up to 8 hours.

Preheat an outdoor grill or a stovetop grill pan to medium-high heat.

Remove the chicken from the marinade (reserving any leftover). Grill the chicken until golden brown and a thermometer inserted in the thickest portion registers 160°F, about 3 minutes per side.

Transfer the leftover marinade to a small saucepan and heat over medium heat. Add the wine and bring to a boil. Reduce to a simmer and cook until the sauce has reduced by half, 5 to 6 minutes. Whisk in the butter until it is completely melted.

Serve the grilled chicken breasts topped with the sauce.

PER SERVING: 365 calories, 31 g protein, 3 g carbohydrates, 24 g total fat (6 g saturated), 98 mg cholesterol, 1 g fiber, 414 mg sodium

- 2 **lemons—1 zested and cut crosswise into ⅛-inch-thick slices, 1 squeezed to yield ¼ cup juice**

  Grated zest of 1 orange
- ¼ **cup olive oil**
- 2 **tablespoons rice vinegar**
- ½ **cup chopped fresh basil, loosely packed**
- ¼ **cup chopped flat-leaf parsley**
- 1 **tablespoon finely chopped garlic**
- 1 **teaspoon finely chopped fresh ginger**
- 1 **teaspoon finely chopped fresh lemongrass**
- 2 **tablespoons lemon-pepper seasoning**
- 6 **bone-in, skin-on free-range organic chicken breast halves**
- ¼ **cup dry white wine**
- 1 **tablespoon unsalted butter**

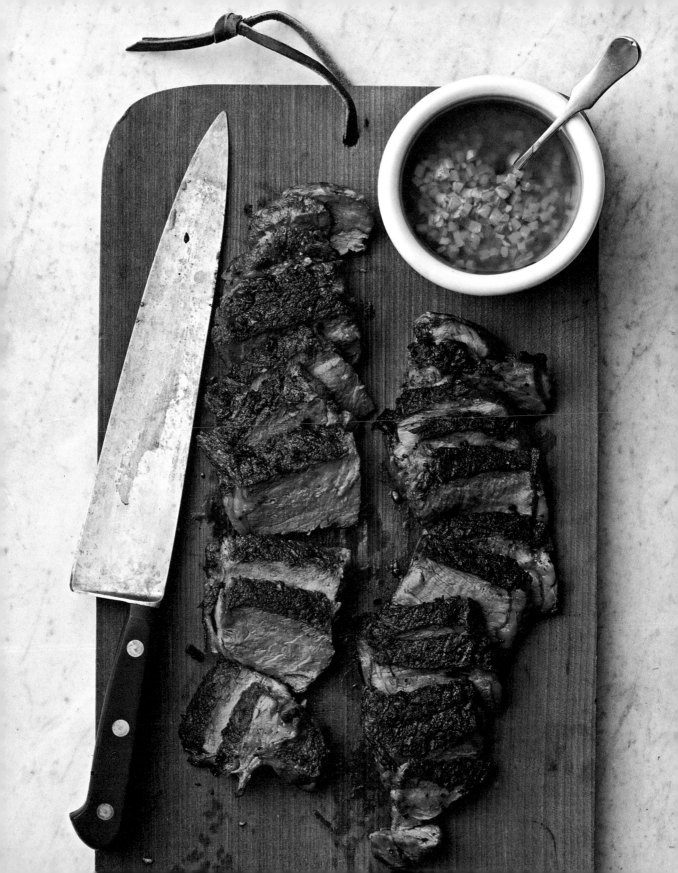

Grilled Strip Loin with Carrot-Ginger Vinaigrette

 4–6 Sliced meat on a slate or marble platter is sexy and sleek. It's very minimal but still seems lavish, with the meat sharply cut and finished with sea salt, the juices running after mixing with the vinaigrette. It looks like it tastes—which is absolutely wonderful.

To make the vinaigrette: In a medium skillet, heat 2 tablespoons of the garlic oil over medium-high heat. Add the carrots, ginger, and garlic and cook until the carrots are fork-tender, 2 to 3 minutes. Remove from the heat and set aside.

In a food processor or blender, combine the onion, vinegar, agave nectar, sambal, soy sauce, mustard, salt, and pepper. Blend the mixture until smooth, gradually adding the remaining ¾ cup plus 2 tablespoons garlic oil in a slow stream. Transfer the mixture to a small bowl and fold in the carrot-ginger mixture. If the vinaigrette is too thick for your liking, stir in 1 teaspoon of cold water. Set aside.

To cook the steaks: In a large bowl, whisk together the garlic oil, rosemary, chopped garlic, shallot, and vinegar. Add the steaks, turning to coat well with the marinade, then set the bowl aside to rest at room temperature for 10 minutes.

Preheat an outdoor grill or a stovetop grill pan to medium-high heat. Grill the steaks without turning for 2 minutes. Rotate them 45 degrees and cook another 2 minutes. Flip them over and repeat. The steaks cook a total of 4 minutes per side for medium-rare.

Transfer the cooked steaks to a cutting board and season to taste with salt and pepper. Let the steaks rest for 3 to 4 minutes before thinly slicing them against the grain. Serve the sliced steak topped with a couple tablespoons of the vinaigrette.

PER SERVING: 373 calories, 40 g protein, 8 g carbohydrates, 20 g total fat (4 g saturated), 91 mg cholesterol, 1 g fiber, 259 mg sodium

CARROT-GINGER VINAIGRETTE

- 1 cup Roasted Garlic Oil (page 93)
- 3 carrots, finely diced
- 3 tablespoons grated ginger
- 2 garlic cloves, finely chopped
- 1 large yellow onion, finely diced
- ½ cup red wine vinegar
- 3 tablespoons agave nectar
- 2 tablespoons sambal oelek chili paste
- 2 tablespoons reduced-sodium soy sauce
- 1 tablespoon Dijon mustard
- ½ teaspoon sea salt
- ¼ teaspoon freshly ground black pepper

STEAK

- 3 tablespoons Roasted Garlic Oil (page 93)
- 3 tablespoons chopped fresh rosemary
- 4 garlic cloves, finely chopped
- 1 shallot, finely diced
- 2 tablespoons red wine vinegar
- 2 strip loin steaks (12 to 14 ounces each), preferably aged
- Salt and freshly ground black pepper

Grilled Skirt Steak with Seared Onion Ponzu

This dish is a great example of the Japanese less-is-more approach to cooking. The ponzu is all the steak needs. The flavors are perfectly balanced and they get love-stoned when combined. I make this dish for parties and serve it sliced, family-style, with the ponzu cascading off the sliced steak. People turn into loiterers and sort of poach from the platter. It's like watching a flock of seagulls hovering. Hilarious. You'll see.

To marinate the steak: In a large bowl, combine the vinegar, garlic oil, ginger, garlic, lemongrass, and agave nectar. Add the steak, turning to coat well in the marinade. Cover the bowl tightly with plastic wrap and refrigerate for at least 4 hours or overnight.

To make the ponzu sauce: Drizzle the onion rings with the oil and sprinkle lightly with salt and black pepper. Heat a medium skillet over medium-high heat until it begins to smoke. Add the onion rings and sear, flipping once, until charred on both sides, 4 to 5 minutes. Let the onion cool in the pan. When cool enough to handle, finely chop and transfer to a small bowl.

Add ⅓ cup cold water, the soy sauce, vinegar, orange juice, lime juice, pineapple juice, agave nectar, garlic oil, scallions, shallots, ginger, and chile. Set aside.

Preheat an outdoor grill or a stovetop grill pan to medium-high heat. Grill the steak for 4 minutes, rotate 45 degrees, and cook for another 4 minutes. Then flip the steak and grill it for another 4 minutes for medium-rare. Transfer the steak to a cutting board and let rest for 3 to 4 minutes before slicing against the grain into ¼-inch-thick strips.

Transfer the sliced steak to a serving platter and serve topped with the ponzu sauce.

PER SERVING: 306 calories, 25 g protein, 15 g carbohydrates, 16 g total fat (4 g saturated), 65 mg cholesterol, 1 g fiber, 464 mg sodium

STEAK

- **2 tablespoons rice vinegar**
- **2 tablespoons Roasted Garlic Oil (page 93)**
- **2 tablespoons grated ginger**
- **2 tablespoon chopped garlic**
- **2 tablespoons finely chopped lemongrass**
- **2 tablespoons agave nectar**
- **1 (2-pound) skirt steak**

PONZU SAUCE

- **1 large yellow onion, cut into ½-inch-thick rings**
- **1 tablespoon olive oil**
- **Salt and freshly ground black pepper**
- **⅓ cup low-sodium soy sauce**
- **3 tablespoons rice vinegar**
- **Juice of 1 orange**
- **Juice of 1 lime**
- **2 tablespoons agave nectar**
- **1 tablespoon Roasted Garlic Oil (page 93)**
- **6 scallions, thinly sliced**
- **2 shallots, diced**
- **3 tablespoons grated ginger**
- **1 serrano chile, thinly sliced**

Espresso-Rubbed Filet Mignon with English Peas

4

It's a story as old as the hills: A redneck from Charleston, South Carolina, moves to New York City, opens up a restaurant, rubs some coffee grounds on a piece of meat, and the rest is history. Okay, it might not have happened exactly that way, but all joking aside, this recipe is one my favorites. I've been making it for almost 10 years now, and every time it works like a charm, fits like a glove, floats like a butterfly, and stings like a bee. By the way, this marinade works great on pork, chicken, and obviously all cuts of beef, so get it done.

Preheat the oven to 400°F.

In a small bowl, mix together the olive oil, honey, espresso, cardamom, cumin, salt, and pepper. Rub the paste onto the steaks until well coated on all sides, then set the steaks aside at room temperature while you make the potatoes and peas.

In a large skillet, heat the butter over medium-high heat. Add the garlic and shallot and cook until translucent. Add the peas and cumin and cook for 1 to 2 minutes. Add the pea shoots and cook just until wilted, about 2 minutes. Remove from the heat and season to taste with salt and pepper.

In a large ovenproof skillet, heat the canola oil over high heat until it begins to smoke. Add the steaks and cooking, without turning, until a crust forms, about 3 minutes. Turn the steaks over and transfer the pan to the oven. Roast until the steaks are medium-rare, about 4 minutes.

Remove the steaks from the oven, transfer to a cutting board, and let rest for 3 to 4 minutes at room temperature before slicing.

To serve, divide the peas among 4 plates, fan the sliced steaks over the vegetables, and sprinkle each serving with the fleur de sel.

PER SERVING: 672 calories, 58 g protein, 25 g carbohydrates, 38 g total fat (12 g saturated), 170 mg cholesterol, 6 g fiber, 489 mg sodium

¼ cup extra-virgin olive oil

1 tablespoon orange blossom honey

3 tablespoons finely ground espresso beans

1½ teaspoons ground cardamom

1 teaspoon ground cumin

1 teaspoon fine sea salt

½ teaspoon freshly ground black pepper

4 filet mignons (½ pound each), preferably aged

2 tablespoons unsalted butter

1 garlic clove, finely chopped

1 shallot, finely diced

2 cups shelled fresh green peas

1 teaspoon ground cumin

1 pound pea shoots

Salt and freshly ground black pepper

1 tablespoon canola oil

1 tablespoon fleur de sel

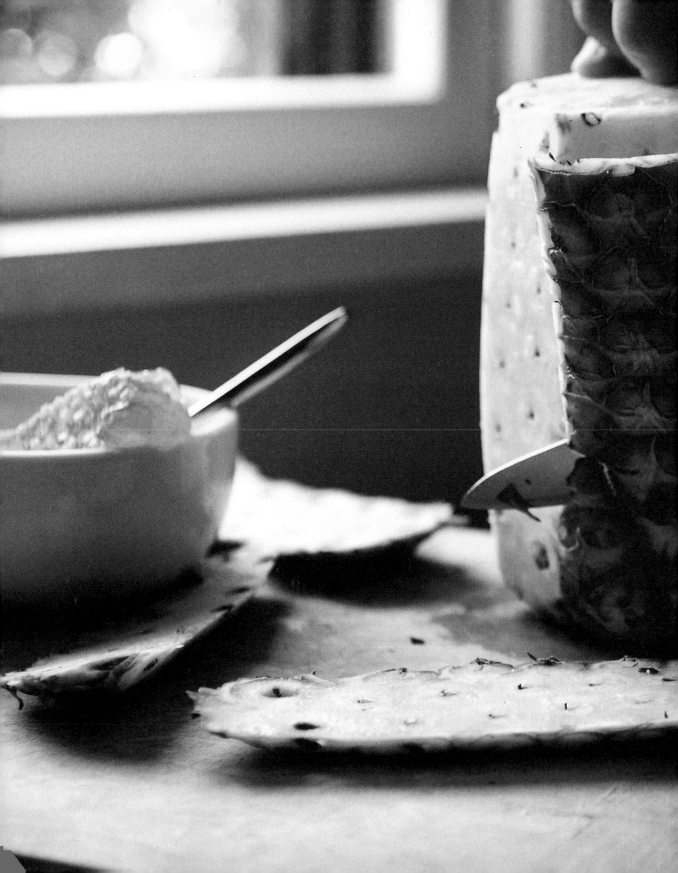

SWEET RESOLUTION

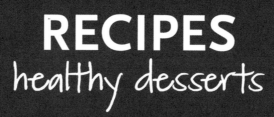

RECIPES
healthy desserts

P rior to my diabetes diagnosis, I wasn't really around sweets all that much. My mom didn't keep a lot of soda and candy around the house; she hadn't grown up with that stuff, so I didn't either. But I had a sweet tooth for sure, and as a young gun hanging out at friends' houses, I would dig into the Oreos, Fruit Loops, M&Ms—all that jackpot stuff—whenever I had the chance.

Once I was diagnosed with diabetes, it was pretty much goodbye to all that over-sugared, saturated-fat-laden junk food. But my sweet tooth didn't go away. Not by a long shot. So what do you do when you have a sweet tooth, and a lot of the sweet things most people eat are essentially off limits—at least most of the time?

You improvise another way to satisfy the urge, that's what. You find substitutes for sugar— I don't have a problem with them if they're natural, like sweeteners derived from the stevia plant. And you use carbohydrate ingredients that are absorbed into the bloodstream more slowly than regular granulated sugar is, so they don't threaten your blood sugar level. As it turns out, there's a world of such sugar substitutes and slow-go carb ingredients. And to a professional chef, they offer an extraordinary opportunity to let my creativity run free and go a little wild. Creativity is always harder when it has to work within some parameters, but working harder tends to make the results better—as you'll see when you try these recipes. Don't think for a second that just because it's not ice cream or cake or some sort of truffle that your ending can't be sweet. I would never let that happen. Granted, it's true that for me cooking is the sweetest thing in my Sweet Life—my daily dessert. But every life deserves a sweet at the end of a day—certainly at the end of a meal—and my aim in these final recipes is to provide sweet endings that are as notable for what they contribute to the body's wellness as for their taste.

OPPOSITES ATTRACT

So is there life after Friendly's? As the saying goes, the proof of the pudding is in the eating. But it all comes down to one word: balance. Living within the parameters diabetes imposes requires balance. And one great way to achieve balance is to create the kind of tension that holds two normally opposing forces together. It may sound like physics, but it's really a matter of taste.

I love mixing things that don't "match." I do it in the way I dress—high-fashion jeans with a faded hoodie and the oldest work boots on earth. It's the way I've furnished my home— part cool contemporary design, part flea market. I like to put old and new together, fancy and plain, light and dark. Ditto in cooking. I like to bring together sweet and pungent, hot and cool, spicy and mild, sharp and gentle. You see it in every chapter and every category of recipe in this book, but I think you see it most of all in these desserts.

Hot chile with the perfume of honey. Cool yogurt with tart ginger. The summer taste of raspberries with the minty edge of fall or winter. Put these things together and what happens? Each enhances the other. Precisely because the yogurt is cool, you can really savor the tartness of the ginger—and vice versa, of course. And the combined taste—the twinned sensation—is something else altogether.

In other words, the balancing of two opposites doesn't dull their power; it makes the power of each emerge. The two tastes resolve into something of their own, just as the disparate tastes in these dessert recipes resolve into a sensation that is so agreeable, so pleasing to the palate, so delightful in its effect that the only word for it is "sweet." That's how you get a sweet resolution. It's one of the great things about cooking.

Alternative Sweeteners

Because refined sugar = carbs = blood sugar spike, I generally look for other options when I need to make something sweet. These are some of the ones I use most:

Agave nectar is very low on the glycemic index, meaning that it won't cause a spike in your blood sugar levels the way sugar does.

Honey is in the same category as agave. It adds just the right amount of sweetness, but it doesn't lead to a spike in blood sugar and will help keep hunger cravings in check.

Stevia extract is made from the leaves of the stevia plant (*Stevia rebaudiana* 'Bertoni'). Stevia has been used in Argentina, Brazil, and Paraguay for centuries to sweeten foods and drinks and is widely cultivated in Asia. While fresh leaves are reported to be 15 to 20 times sweeter than sugar, extracts from the leaves are 250 to 300 times sweeter. In granulated

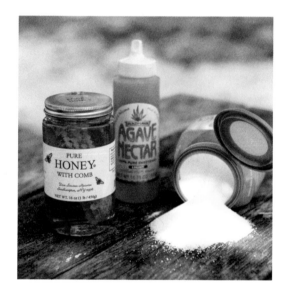

form, the sweetness can vary from brand to brand, so check the label for guidelines when replacing sugar in recipes.

NUTRITION AND WELLNESS

I also promise wellness and nutritional benefits in these desserts, and it's a promise that's important to keep. The truth is, the sweetest of resolutions comes with the healthiest of ingredients.

For example, many of these desserts feature fruits that are low on the glycemic index: pears and peaches and apples each have a GI ranking of 38, strawberries are at 40, mango and banana 51 and 52, respectively. These fruits are all high in fiber—particularly those with edible skins like apples—and fiber really puts a brake on the speed with which sugar is absorbed into the bloodstream. Several of these fruits—apples, pears, and mangoes in particular—are high-fructose foods; more specifically, they contain a high fructose-to-glucose ratio. This is a good thing because fructose metabolizes without the use of insulin, so it's an easy way for diabetics to get the health benefits, not to mention the sweet taste, of fruit—whether it's fresh, frozen, or canned.

In a sense, everything I know about health and taste—everything I care about in terms of my life and my profession—more or less comes together in these desserts. Take, for example, the Sour Strawberry Cobbler (page 229). Strawberries are so common these days that we are likely to take them for granted. Find them in jams, jellies, syrups, confections, and of course raw, where their deep red color is a signal of their phenomenal phytonutrient content.

The health benefits of strawberries? Start with eye health, which the rich antioxidant content of strawberries does battle for. Ditto for the prevention of degeneration of muscles and tissues—as in arthritis, for example—for strawberries are also rich in detoxifiers; in India, the saying is that a serving of strawberries can remove the rust from the joints. These same detoxifiers and antioxidants also fight cancer, support brain function, lower high blood pressure, and are great for the cardiovascular system.

But what my Sour Strawberry Cobbler is really about is reclaiming the essence of cobblers. They've been overtaken in recent years by a single, cookie-cutter, sugary version that has become standard. The cobbler recipe here embraces the spirit of a dessert—something yummy to wrap up a meal—without the crazy blood sugar spikes and mood swings of those degraded contemporary saccharine cobblers. I use the word "sour" as a suggestion rather than a description. What you're going to taste here is strawberry—rich and richly nutritious, piquant and enlivening, and in the truest sense of the word, a perfectly *sweet* resolution of good health and good eating.

All Fruits Are Not Created Equal

While all fruits clock in relatively high on the glycolic index compared to most vegetables, eaten in moderation they can absolutely be on the menu every day if you want. That said, it's good to know where your favorites rank. I hate to admit it, but one of my all-time faves, watermelon, is way up there, as are dates, with a rating of nearly 100 compared to an apple at 38 or a plum at 24. However, watermelon's glycemic *load* is relatively low. Either way, keep an eye on portion control when choosing a fruit, and make sure it's really fresh and delicious (otherwise, why bother?).

LOW GI (55 OR BELOW)

When I really need fruit fix, I usually go for the freshest apples I can get my hands on; they have one of the lowest GIs of any fruit. Oranges, pears, fresh peaches and strawberries are also great alternatives.

MEDIUM (56 TO 69)

Pineapples, mangoes, bananas, and papayas are a bit higher on the index; I don't mind reaching for one of these when I feel like I'm about to encounter low blood sugar or just need a boost.

HIGH (70 AND OVER)

Watermelon, dates

The Mighty Mango

A king among fruits, the mango is so packed with nutrients of every sort it is virtually a pharmacy package, so it's little wonder that it has long been used as a traditional remedy—thought by some to have magical properties—for any number of ailments. Amino acids, vitamins C and E, flavonoids, beta-carotene, niacin, calcium, iron, magnesium, potassium: Mangoes are packed with these vitamins, minerals, and phytonutrients. What can they do for you? Fight cancer, for one thing, especially cancers of the gastrointestinal tract. Promote eyesight—thanks to the mango's beta-carotene content—plus keep the eyes moist and comfortable. Aid digestion—and calm a rough stomach if you have one. Improve your complexion (use the pulp to unclog pores). Boost your memory. Treat anemia—mangoes are a sweet way to add iron to the system. Charge your sex drive. Really.

One more thing: Mangoes are great in fighting diabetes. The leaves help normalize insulin levels, so an infusion made from the leaves is a great cup of tea for diabetics. And, of course, with its low glycemic level, chowing down chunks of the golden, luscious fruit is a wonderful (and delicious) way to take in needed fiber.

And what can one say about the taste of mango? Taste is so subjective that trying to pin it down is like trying to describe being in love. Actually, eating a ripe mango is almost as exciting as being in love, and it offers a similar combination of mellow sweetness and a hint of an edge.

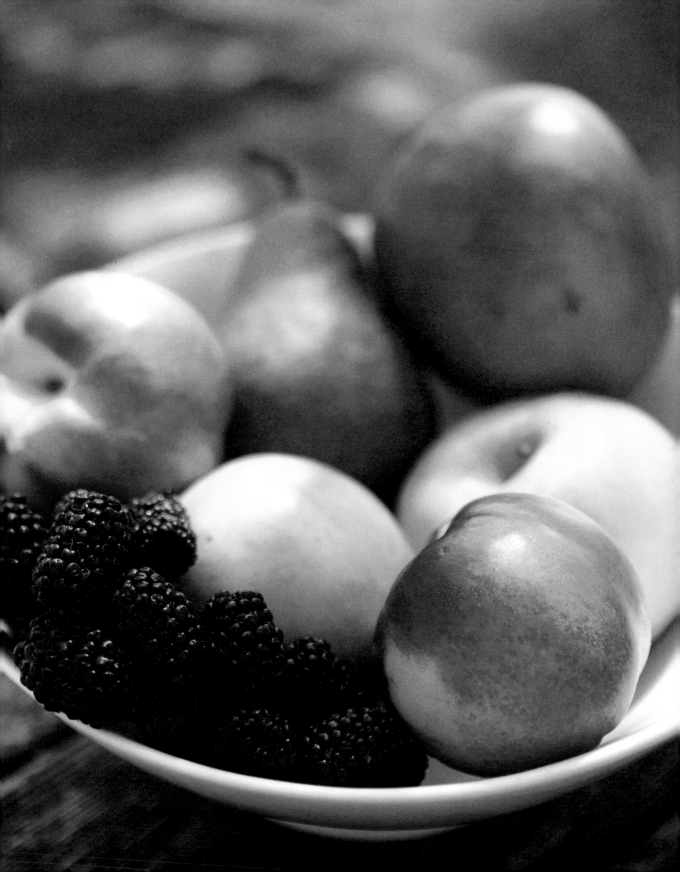

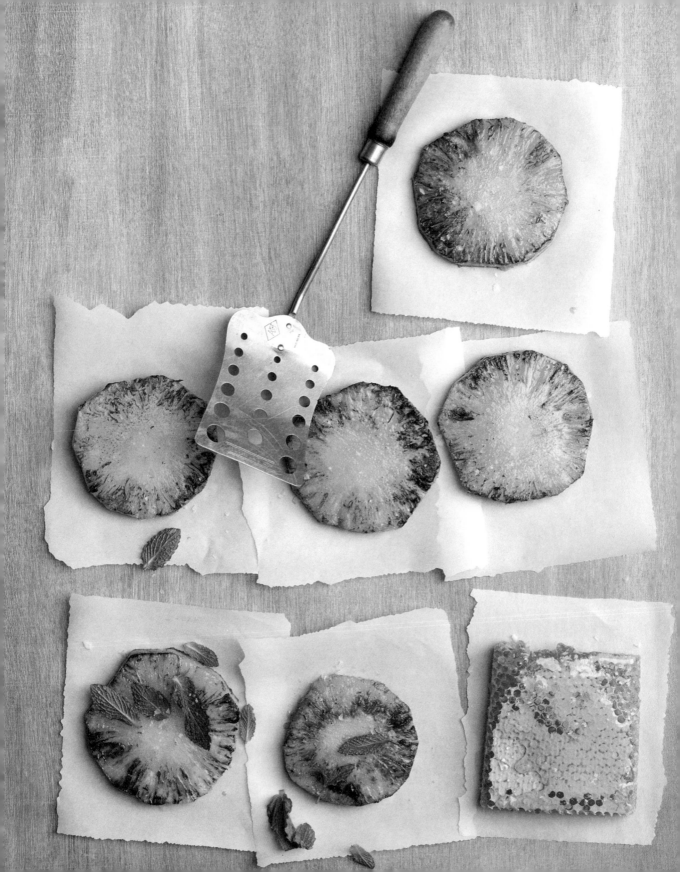

Charred Pineapple with Honeycomb

 6

Colombia is one of the most charming countries I've visited, with crazy landscapes and mountain views that can bring you to your knees. They also grow the most amazing giant pineapples vibrant yellow, and beyond sweet—sun-ripened and succulent. Closer to home, farmstands along the side of the road on the way to Montauk sell freshly peeled pineapple chunks on a stick or by the plastic bagful; I may have hoped for a low blood sugar while driving by so I could OD on the fresh *piña*!

Use a sharp, large knife to cut off the pineapple rind. Cut crosswise into 6 ½-inch-thick slices (save the rest for another use). In a large skillet, heat the butter over high heat. When the butter begins to bubble, add the pineapple and cook without turning until the sugars start to caramelize, 1 to 2 minutes.

Turn gently with tongs and cook until the pineapple has a nice golden color on all sides, 2 to 3 minutes. Transfer the pineapple to a platter and sprinkle with the mint and sea salt.

Top each round with a teaspoon of honeycomb.

- 1 **pineapple, small**
- 1 **tablespoon butter**
- ½ **cup hand-torn fresh mint leaves**
- ½ **teaspoon coarse sea salt**
- 6 **teaspoon-size scoops honeycomb**

PER SERVING: 45 calories, 1 g protein, 7 g carbohydrates, 2 g total fat (1 g saturated), 5 mg cholesterol, 1 g fiber, 139 mg sodium

Warm Mango with Chile Agave

 This recipe brings it all up front—the sweetness and the spice, the array of tastes, colors, and textures—opposites embracing each other and enhancing each other. It's all about balance, and that's the key to the Sweet Life.

To make the chile honey: In a blender, combine the lime zest and juice, agave nectar, chili paste, and ¼ cup water. Blend on a low setting until smooth.

To cook the mangoes: In a large skillet, melt the butter over medium-high heat. When the butter begins to bubble, add the mangoes and cook without stirring for 30 seconds. Stir in the coconut milk and mint.

Transfer the mango mixture to a serving platter. Serve with the chile honey drizzled over the top.

PER SERVING: 130 calories, 1 g protein, 26 g carbohydrates, 4 g total fat (3 g saturated), 5 mg cholesterol, 2 g fiber, 15 mg sodium

CHILE AGAVE

Grated zest and juice of 3 limes

2 tablespoons agave nectar

½ teaspoon chili paste (sambal oelek)

MANGO

1 tablespoon unsalted butter

3 mangoes, diced

¼ cup coconut milk

¼ cup loosely packed hand-torn fresh mint leaves

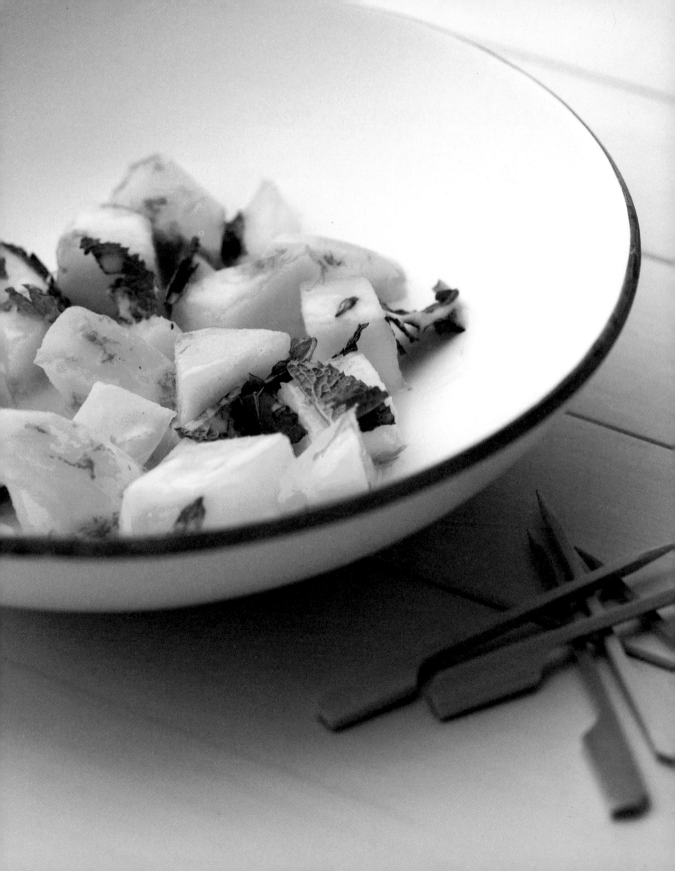

Lavender Poached Pears

 Making this dessert puts you instantly in the best mood because it smells so damn good, and the combined essences of the fresh and dried herbs perfume the dish in a very sensual way. The pear, which can be very sweet on its own, might seem timid against the lavender, but they complement each other really well. It's an exciting combination of flavors you normally don't see paired together. I usually use Bosc pears, but you can use any variety that is in season.

Peel, halve, and core the pears using a melon baller to scoop out the seeds.

In a large pot, combine 3 cups water, the sweetener, lavender, hibiscus, chamomile tea, and mint. Bring to a boil over medium-high heat, then reduce the heat to medium-low, add the pears, and simmer until you can easily pierce the pears with the tip of a knife, about 20 minutes.

To serve, transfer the pear halves to 4 individual bowls and ladle some of the cooking liquid over the top.

2 **large ripe Bosc pears, slightly firm to the touch**

3 **tablespoons granulated stevia extract, or to taste**

1 **tablespoon dried lavender**

2 **blossoms dried hibiscus**

1 **chamomile tea bag**

½ **cup loosely packed fresh mint leaves**

PER SERVING: 72 calories, 1 g protein, 19 g carbohydrates, 0 g total fat (0 g saturated), 0 mg cholesterol, 4 g fiber, 2 mg sodium

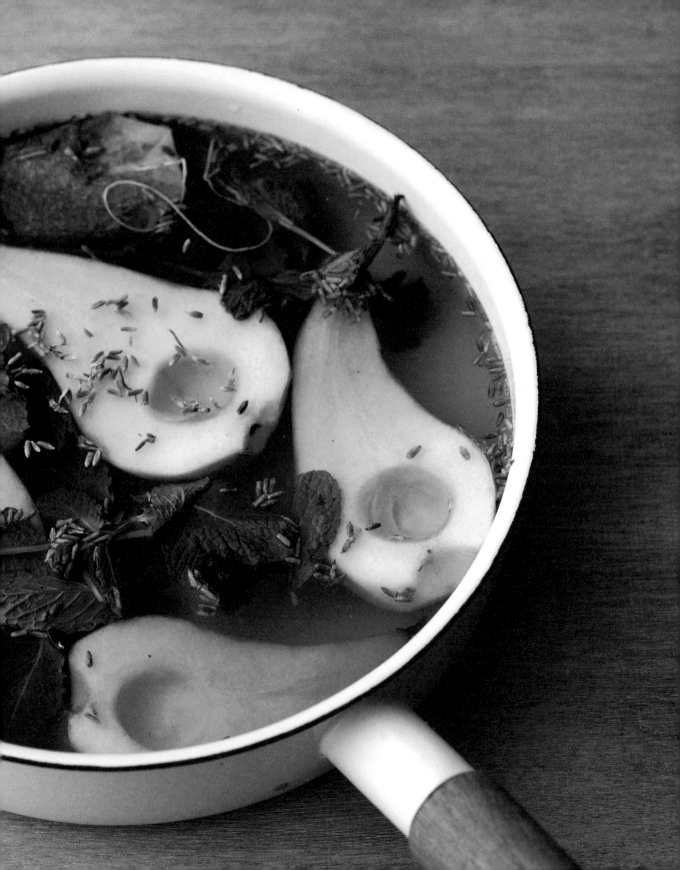

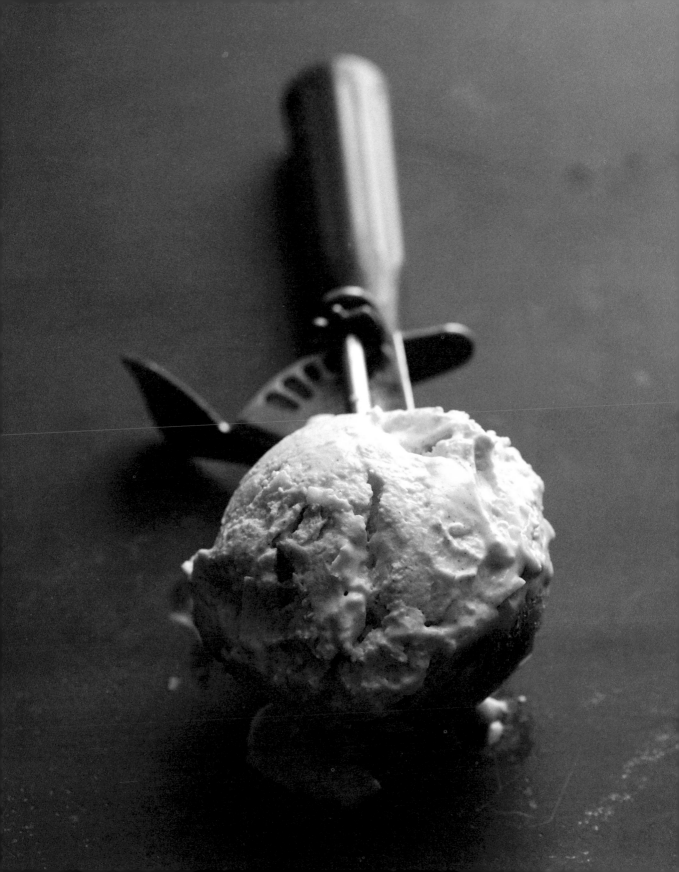

Frozen Coconut Yogurt with Cinnamon

 6–8

Frozen yogurt! I mean let's face it: Everybody loves a good frozen yogurt. Adults, tweens, teens, kids, whoever. You've seen it a hundred times at your local ice cream parlor on Sunday in the summer: 9:00 p.m. and the place is packed! A line around the corner, kids playing, everybody's happy; it's the sweet life. For a diabetic, that could go two ways: One way is horribly wrong, and that's if there're no sugar-free items on the board. Or, totally great because they do offer some special items for people with some sort of dietary restriction. Or there's Plan C, which is that you make a batch of this silky, creamy, coconut yogurt at home and relax with the fam on Sunday night. Let the others rush to the corner store and wait in line; your only fear will be whether or not your family leaves you any.

In a large bowl, combine the yogurt, sweetener, coconut milk, cinnamon, and coconut extract. Cover tightly with plastic wrap and let the mixture chill in the fridge for at least 1 hour or overnight.

Pour the chilled mixture into an ice cream maker and freeze according to the manufacturer's instructions for frozen yogurt. In the last 5 minutes of the maker's cycle, add the shredded coconut.

PER SERVING: 80 calories, 1 g protein, 17 g carbohydrates, 6 g total fat (5 g saturated), 0 mg cholesterol, 1 g fiber, 3 mg sodium

3 cups 2% plain organic Greek yogurt

Granulated stevia extract equivalent to ½ cup sugar

2 tablespoons coconut milk

1 teaspoon ground cinnamon

1 teaspoon coconut extract

½ cup unsweetened shredded coconut

Spiced Roasted Apples with Almonds

4

The flavors in this easy dessert remind me of fall and it would be perfect as part of a Thanksgiving spread. The smell of the apples along with the aromatic spices slow cooking in the pan is irresistible.

Toast the nuts in a medium, heavy-bottomed skillet over medium-high heat for 3 to 4 minutes, or until golden. Remove to a plate and set aside to cool. Wipe out the skillet.

In the same skillet, combine the agave, cinnamon, and nutmeg with ¼ cup of water. Cook over medium heat, stirring often, until the agave dissolves and the mixture bubbles.

Add the apples to the pan and stir to coat in the agave mixture. Cook, turning often, for 8 to 10 minutes or until the apples are tender. Spoon into serving bowls and drizzle with a bit of the syrup. Top with a tablespoon of yogurt and sprinkle with the toasted almonds.

½ **cup almonds, roughly chopped**

¼ **cup agave nectar**

½ **teaspoon of cinnamon**

¼ **teaspoon ground nutmeg**

2 **large Golden Delicious apples, peeled, cored, and sliced in 8ths**

¼ **cup plain Greek yogurt**

PER SERVING: 219 calories, 5 g protein, 30 g carbohydrates, 11 g total fat (2 g saturated), 3 mg cholesterol, 3 g fiber, 6 mg sodium

Key Lime Pie

If you can get fresh key limes (they are in season in the late winter months), go for it; the rest of the year, though, bottled key lime juice works just fine, making this a year-round favorite. Serve topped with a little extra whipped cream if you like, or just as is.

To make the crust: Place the bran cereal and graham cracker crumbs in a food processor and pulse to make fine crumbs. With the processor running, add 5 to 6 tablespoons of cold water; the crumbs should be moist but not damp. Spray a 9-inch pie pan with nonstick cooking spray and turn the crumbs into the pan. Press the crumbs onto the bottom and sides of the pan to make a thin crust. Chill.

To make the filling: Combine the lime juice and zest in a small saucepan and heat until warm. Whisk in the gelatin until completely dissolved, then set aside to cool to room temperature. Beat the cream cheese with an electric mixer until smooth. Beat in 6 tablespoons of the sweetener, then stir in the cooled lime juice mixture. Place the mixing bowl in a larger bowl filled with ice and water and stir with a rubber spatula until thickened; the texture should be similar to a custard. Set aside.

In a separate bowl beat the cream and agave syrup with the remaining 2 tablespoons of sweetener until stiff. Fold a scoop of the whipped cream into the cream cheese mixture to lighten it, then fold in the remaining whipped cream, mixing until fairly well combined (it doesn't have to be completely incorporated.

Pour the filling into the prepared crust and smooth the top. Refrigerate for 3 to 4 hours, or until firm enough to cut into wedges. Garnish with fresh fruit or mint.

PER SERVING: 262 calories, 4 g protein, 16 g carbohydrates, 21 g total fat (13 g saturated), 71 mg cholesterol, 1 g fiber, 153 mg sodium

CRUST
- ½ cup All-Bran cereal
- ½ cup graham cracker crumbs

FILLING
- ½ cup key lime juice (the bottled kind works well)
- ¼ teaspoon grated lime zest
- 1 packet (2 teaspoons) unflavored gelatin
- 8 ounces cream cheese, at room temperature
- Granulated stevia extract equivalent to ¾ cup sugar
- 1 cup heavy cream
- 1 tablespoon agave syrup
- Fresh fruit or mint leaves for garnish

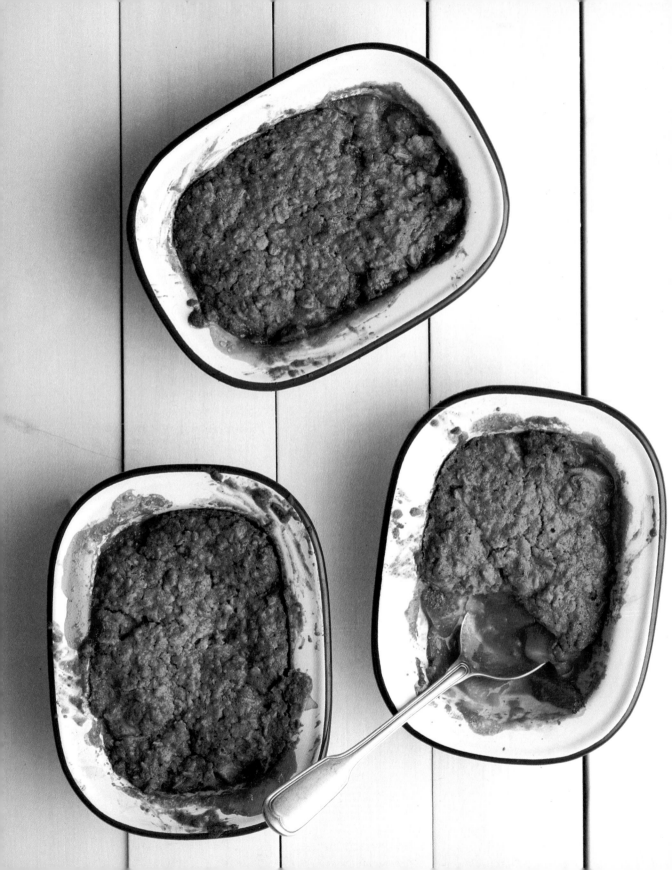

Sour Strawberry Cobbler

Tart is the word of the day here. I'm so sick of the oversweetened, overcompensated, thick, fatty cobblers that taste of just sugar and butter so many bakeries and chefs seem to be turning out lately. I actually like to be able to taste the fruit that was supposed to take the leading role in a cobbler—before sugar kicked its ass. For this cobbler, I use fresh strawberries and only when they're in season. Strawberries in January taste like cardboard. Wait till summer and try to get your hands on some local berries; it's well worth the wait. I tweak the dish by adding some fresh lime juice to heighten the flavor and offer a real sense of refreshment. It's such a small amount that you hardly notice it, but when you do, you'll be much obliged—I hope. Another cool chef's trick to try if you have time: I like to freeze half the sliced strawberries overnight, then stir them into the fruit mixture just before baking; I think it brings out even more of their sweetness.

To make the filling: In a large bowl, combine the strawberries with the oat flour, sweetener, agave nectar, and lime zest and juice.

Preheat the oven to 375°F. Butter the bottom and sides of a 2-quart baking dish.

To make the topping: In a large bowl, using your fingertips, combine the rolled oats, oat flour, baking powder, sweetener, cinnamon, and butter. Add the almond milk and agave nectar and continue mixing with your fingertips until a rough dough forms.

Pour the filling into the prepared baking dish and spoon on the topping. Transfer the baking dish to the oven and bake the cobbler until golden brown and bubbly, 35 to 40 minutes.

PER SERVING: 243 calories, 4 g protein, 29 g carbohydrates, 13 g total fat (7 g saturated), 31 mg cholesterol, 4 g fiber, 195 mg sodium

FILLING

- 2 pints thinly sliced strawberries
- ½ cup oat flour
- 3 tablespoons granulated stevia extract, or to taste
- 1 tablespoon agave nectar
- Grated zest of 1 lime and juice of 3 limes

TOPPING

- 1 cup old-fashioned rolled oats
- ½ cup oat flour
- 1 tablespoon baking powder
- 1 teaspoon ground cinnamon
- 8 tablespoons (1 stick) unsalted butter, cut into small pieces
- ½ cup almond milk
- 3 tablespoons agave nectar

Peanut Butter and Oatmeal Cookies

 A hybrid of my two childhood favorites—peanut butter cookies and oatmeal raisin—these couldn't be easier to throw together. They store really well for up to a week, so don't eat them all at once; even though they are relatively low in carbs compared to their white-flour cousins, they still should be considered a once-in-awhile treat at 20 grams of carbs apiece.

Preheat the oven to 350°F. Grease a large baking sheet.

In a mixing bowl, combine the peanut butter, sweetener, eggs, oats, and vanilla and stir with a rubber spatula to make a stiff dough. Roll the dough into balls the size of large cherries and arrange on the baking sheet, 2 inches apart.

With a fork, flatten the cookies, turning the tines 90 degrees to create a crisscross pattern and dipping the tines in a bit of additional sweetener each time to prevent sticking.

Bake for 12 minutes, then remove from the oven and sprinkle the cookies with a bit of cinnamon. Let the cookies cool completely on the baking sheets. Store in an airtight container for up to a week.

1 cup creamy peanut butter

Granulated stevia extract equivalent to ¾ cup of sugar

2 eggs

½ cup quick oats

2 teaspoon pure vanilla extract

Cinnamon for garnish

PER COOKIE: 126 calories, 5 g protein, 8 g carbohydrates, 9 g total fat (2 g saturated), 23 mg cholesterol, 1 g fiber, 82 mg sodium

Spiced Sesame Oranges

When unexpected guests show up for dinner, this is the kind of dessert you can whip together in a few minutes out of things you probably have on your pantry shelf. Play around with the spices if you like; if allspice jumps out at you, that would be great, too, and you can use tangerines or tangelos instead of the oranges. Don't let the fruit sit too long though or it will start to break down.

Using a sharp knife, slice off the orange skins removing all the pith and catching any juices on a plate. Slice the oranges crosswise into 5 or 6 slices and place in a shallow bowl.

In a small bowl stir together the honey, vanilla, cinnamon, and sesame seeds, along with the collected juice and mix until combined. Drizzle over the orange slices. Chill for up to to 45 minutes. Serve the spiced citrus slices topped with the cream or goat cheese, and drizzle some of the sauce over each portion.

PER SERVING: 197 calories, 2 g protein, 20 g carbohydrates, 13 g total fat (7 g saturated), 41 mg cholesterol, 2 g fiber, 14 mg sodium

- **2 large navel oranges**
- **2 tablespoons honey**
- **1 teaspoon vanilla extract**
- **$\frac{1}{2}$ teaspoon ground cinnamon**
- **$\frac{1}{2}$ tablespoon black sesame seeds**
- **$\frac{1}{2}$ tablespoon white sesame seeds**
- **$\frac{1}{2}$ cup heavy cream, whipped, or $\frac{1}{2}$ cup crumbled soft goat cheese**

ACKNOWLEDGMENTS

For their help in making the experience of creating The Sweet Life so sweet, my thanks go to the following people:

Sam Nato and Joe Abraham, for their Creative Intuitions.

Susanna Margolis, for helping me get the ins and outs of my sweet life down on paper; Peggy Paul also provided assistance in fine-tuning the recipes. Dr. Jason Baker and Eric Ripert were strong believers in my message that food and diabetes can happily coexist in the kitchen and I appreciate their contributions and support.

My Brother from Another, believer, advisor Matty Young, for always having the diginity and strength to keep doing it, and doing it well. Much love.

Everyone responsible for the food-and-fun photos: photographers Tara Donne, Sarah Kehoe, and Joe Termini; creative director Emily Anderson; food stylist Maggie Ruggiero; and prop stylist Harry Bailey.

My restaurant crews at Mondrian Soho Hotel's Imperial No. Nine and the Surf Lodge: Without each and every one of you, none of this would be possible! My special appreciation goes to all of the hard-working mothers both front-of-house and in the kitchen—more power to 'em.

The team at Rodale: fellow surfer and publisher Karen Rinaldi; my editor Pam Krauss; designer Kara Plikaitis; publicist Emily Weber; and Nancy N. Bailey, JoAnn Brader, Tory Glerum, and Aniella Perold.

The *Top Chef* team and Tom, Padma, and Gail.

For all-around guidance and support, a big shout-out to Joel Menzin, Andy Gershon, Jay Strell, Bob Levine, Kim Schefler, Geoff Menin, Nantane Boudreau, Jacob Cooper, Amy Dunn, Michael Principe, Steve Peterson, Jasa Joesph, Yousef Ghalaini, Diane Abraham, the Termini family, Rob McKinley, Tonia Dangelo, and Richard Young.

And lastly Montauk, Charleston, Charlotte, and NYC—I love you all!

INDEX

Underscored page references indicate sidebars and tables. **Boldface** references indicate photographs.